Diagnostic Imaging
of AIDS

Diagnostic Imaging of AIDS

Edited by J. W. A. J. Reeders

Coeditors: F. H. Barneveld Binkhuysen and
J. F. W. M. Bartelsman

with contributions by

H. R. Antonides
F. H. Barneveld Binkhuysen
J. F. W. M. Bartelsman
P. J. E. Bindels
C. A. B. Boucher
P. J. van den Broek
R. A. Coutinho
S. A. Danner
J. A. Dol
J. Goudsmit

P. A. Koster
A. J. Megibow
P. Portegies
J. W. A. J. Reeders
E. A. van Royen
M. E. I. Schipper
R. P. van Steenwijk
J. G. van den Tweel
J. Valk

Forewords by G. W. Stevenson and G. N. J. Tytgat

178 illustrations

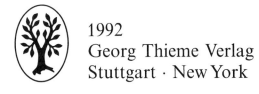

1992
Georg Thieme Verlag   Thieme Medical Publishers, Inc.
Stuttgart · New York   New York

Library of Congress Cataloging-in-Publication Data

Diagnostic imaging of AIDS / edited by
J. W. A. J. Reeders, ; coeditors.
  F. H. Barneveld Binkhuysen and
  J. F. W. N. Bartelsman ; with contributions by
  H. R. Antonides ... [et al.] ; forewords by
  G. W. Stevenson and G. N. J. Tytgat.
      p. cm.
    Includes bibliographical references and index.
    1. AIDS (Disease) – Imaging. I. Reeders,
    Jacques W. A. J.
    II. Barneveld Binkhuysen, F. H. (Frits H.)
    III. Bartelsman, J. F. W. M. (Joep F. W. M.)
    IV. Antonides, H. R. (Herman R.)
      [DNLM: 1. Acquired Immunodeficiency
      Syndrome – diagnosis.
    2. Central Nervous System Diseases – diagnosis.
    3. Diagnostic Imaging. 4. Gastrointestinal
    Diseases – diagnosis. 5. Lung Disease –
    diagnosis. WD 308 D538]
    RC607, A26 D53 1991
    818.97'920751 – dc 20'
    DNLM/DLC
    for Library of Congress   91-34587 CIP

© 1992 Georg Thieme Verlag,
Rüdigerstraße 14, D-7000 Stuttgart 30
Thieme Medical Publishers, Inc., 381 Park Avenue
South, New York, N.Y. 10016

Typesetting by Fotosatz-Service KÖHLER,
D-8700 Würzburg

Printed in Germany by K. Grammlich,
D-7401 Pliezhausen

ISBN 3-13-767001-2 (GTV, Stuttgart)
ISBN 0-86577-416-1 (TMP, New York)

1 2 3 4 5 6

Important Note: Medicine is an ever-changing science undergoing continual development. Research and clinical experience are continually expanding our knowledge, in particular our knowledge of proper treatment and drug therapy. Insofar as this book mentions any dosage or application, readers may rest assured that the authors, editors and publishers have made every effort to ensure that such references are in accordance with the state of knowledge at the time of production of the book.

Nevertheless this does not involve, imply, or express any guarantee or responsibility on the part of the publishers in respect of any dosage instructions and forms of application stated in the book. Every user is requested to examine carefully the manufacturers' leaflets accompanying each drug and to check, if necessary in consultation with a physician or specialist, whether the dosage schedules mentioned therein or the contraindications stated by the manufacturers differ from the statements made in the present book. Such examination is particularly important with drugs that are either rarely used or have been newly released on the market. Every dosage schedule or every form of application used is entirely at the user's own risk and responsibility. The authors and publishers request every user to report to the publishers any discrepancies or inaccuracies noticed.

Foreword

While the AIDS pandemic appears to slow its rate of growth as it spreads into the heterosexual population of the industrial world, it is becoming apparent that the disease is going to dominate many aspects of medical practice for several decades to come.

Radiologists will need to recognize its appearances, to understand how, safely, to look after patients with the disease, and to know enough about the illness to be able to counsel their patients, their staff, and their colleagues. This book from the Netherlands, with contributions from New York, accomplishes these goals admirably.

It is divided into four sections, the first of which provides up-to-date information on the disease, its epidemiology, and its pathophysiology, as well as a chapter on how to prevent transmission in the radiology department.

The other three sections describe the clinical and imaging aspects of the disease in the nervous system, the lungs, and the gastrointestinal tract.

The book has a global approach, including data from Europe, North America, and Africa, and the imaging represents both the European and North American experience.

The book is hard to put down, as it is so well written and the subject matter so urgent. The radiology material is thorough and well illustrated. This book should serve as a reference for radiologists the world over, gathering in one volume a great deal of material that would otherwise require researching a large number of textbooks and journals. The authors have produced a cohesive account of AIDS that will educate and guide radiologic practice.

G. W. Stevenson, FRCP, FRCR, FRCP(C)
Professor and Chairman,
Department of Radiology,
McMaster University Faculty of Health
Sciences
Hamilton, Canada

Head of Section,
Department of Radiology and Nuclear
Medicine,
Chedoke-McMaster Hospitals,
Hamilton, Canada

Foreword

AIDS is currently "the" most devastating illness. Because of its widespread occurrence, any physician in any discipline may be confronted with this disease, its infectious consequences, and its multiorgan involvement, in particular the lung, GI tract, and central nervous system. Especially the gastrointestinal tract and the lungs provide an extensive and intimate interface between the body and the external environment. A variety of immunologic defects may compromise the integrity of the intestinal defense system, resulting in local and systemic infections with otherwise nonpathogenic opportunistic organisms or with more virulent traditional pathogens.

Evaluation of various diseases in patients infected with human immunodeficiency virus (HIV) and in patients with the acquired immune deficiency syndrome (AIDS) became of major clinical importance during the past decade. Because of the dramatic increase in the prevalence of AIDS-related problems in clinical practice, which allowed rapid gathering of knowledge, especially with respect to diagnosis it seemed timely to review all imaging aspects of the AIDS manifestations in the human body.

This monograph sets out to review coherently the current knowledge about the wide range of manifestations in AIDS and accomplishes this in a delightfully readable manner. Moreover, the editors of this monograph on imaging in AIDS have succeeded admirably in bringing together a wealth of information and knowledge through combination of the various leading imaging disciplines. They have achieved a free-flowing uniformity of style. Well-selected and -designed figures and graphs are used freely to illustrate important points. In addition, there is a rich undercurrent of personal experience with the investigations described.

The editors are to be congratulated on producing a book that overcomes the unnecessary rivalry that all too often exists between various imaging techniques. Where appropriate, any technique is given equal prominence in this book.

The intention of this monograph was to evaluate the diagnostic usefulness of the imaging techniques to enable the novice to recognize the abnormalities commonly encountered in AIDS. Indeed, this monograph should be most useful as a guide in the encounter with AIDS patients in daily clinical practice. On the whole it succeeds admirably on this account.

Guido N. J. Tytgat, M. D.
Professor and Chairman,
Department of Gastroenterology,
Academic Medical Center,
Amsterdam

Preface

During the last few years, organ diagnostics in AIDS has gained increasing interest. The aim of this book is to give the radiologist and the clinician treating the patient a clear insight into what radiologic and endoscopic research currently have to offer with regard to AIDS.

This book is a collaboration of representatives from a broad range of medical disciplines (internal medicine, gastroenterology, neurology, radiology, and pathology) at the Academic Medical Center in Amsterdam. It has been designed to give each discipline a chance to contribute – in harmony with the others. In many areas of medicine, including this one, different diagnostic modalities can complement each other.

In addition to revision of basic knowledge, attention is also paid to new developments in radiology, epidemiology, virology, clinical diagnostics, and gastroenterologic manifestations. The danger of infection via diagnostic procedures will be discussed from the practical point of view.

We hope this book will help physicians become more familiar with the radiologic and endoscopic images that can occur in AIDS, and that a responsible choice will be made from the range of possible imaging modalities used in AIDS cases.

In closing, we would like to thank Mrs. B. S. Vollers-King for her translation of the Dutch manuscripts.

We would also like to thank the Dept. of Photography (Head: R. E. Verhoeven) for the high quality images of this book.

J. W. A. J. Reeders
F. H. Barneveld Binkhuysen
J. W. F. M. Bartelsman

Contributors' Adresses

Hermien R. Antonides, M. D.
Department of Radiology
Hospital "Zonnegloren"
Soesterbergsestraatweg 125
3768 MC Soest
The Netherlands

Frits H. Barneveld Binkhuysen, M. D., Ph. D.
Department of Thoracic Radiology
Academic Medical Center
Meibergdreef 9
1105 AZ Amsterdam zuidoost
The Netherlands

Joep F. W. M. Bartelsman, M. D.
Department of Gastroenterology
Academic Medical Center
Meibergdreef 9
1105 AZ Amsterdam zuidoost
The Netherlands

Patrick J. E. Bindels, M. D.
Municipal Health Service
Department of Public Health
Nieuwe Achtergracht 100
Postbus 20244
1000 HE Amsterdam
The Netherlands

Charles A. B. Boucher, M. D.
Department of Microbiology
Human Retrovirus Laboratory
Academic Medical Center
Meibergdreef 9
1105 AZ Amsterdam zuidoost
The Netherlands

Pieter J. van den Broek, M. D., Ph.D.
Department of Internal Medicine
(Infectious Diseases)
Academic Hospital Leiden
Postbus 9600
2300 RC Leiden
The Netherlands

Roeland A. Coutinho, M. D., Ph. D.
Head, Municipal Health Services
Department of Public Health
Nieuwe Achtergracht 100
Postbus 20244
1000 HE Amsterdam
The Netherlands

Sven A. Danner, M. D., Ph. D.
Head, AIDS Clinics
Department of Internal Medicine
Academic Medical Center
Meibergdreef 9
1105 AZ Amsterdam zuidoost
The Netherlands

Johan A. Dol, M. D.
Department of Radiology
Academic Medical Center
Meibergdreef 9
1105 AZ Amsterdam zuidoost
The Netherlands

J. Goudsmit, M. D., Ph. D.
Professor and Chairman
Department of Microbiology
Human Retrovirus Laboratory
Academic Medical Center
Meibergdreef 9
1105 AZ Amsterdam zuidoost
The Netherlands

Pieter A. Koster, M. D.
Department of Neuroradiology
Academic Medical Center
Meibergdreef 9
1105 AZ Amsterdam zuidoost
The Netherlands

Alec J. Megibow, M. D., Professor,
Department of Radiology
New York University Medical Center
560 First Avenue
New York, NY 10016
USA

Peter Portegies, M. D.
Department of Neurology
Academic Medical Center
Meibergdreef 9
1105 AZ Amsterdam zuidoost
The Netherlands

Jacques W. A. J. Reeders, M. D., Ph. D.
Head, Division of GI-Radiology
Academic Medical Center
Meibergdreef 9
1105 AZ Amsterdam zuidoost
The Netherlands

Eric A. van Royen, M. D., Ph. D.
Chairman, Department of Nuclear Medicine
Academic Medical Center
Meibergdreef 9
1105 AZ Amsterdam zuidoost
The Netherlands

Margarithe E. I. Schipper, M. D.
Department of Pathology
Onze Lieve Vrouwe Gasthuis
1ᵉ Oosterparkstraat 179
1091 HA, Amsterdam
The Netherlands

Reindert P. van Steenwijk, M. D., Ph. D.
Department of Pulmonology
Academic Medical Center
Amsterdam
The Netherlands

Jan G. van den Tweel, M. D., Ph. D.
Professor and Chairman,
Department of Pathology
University Hospital Utrecht
Heidelberglaan 100
3584 CX Utrecht
The Netherlands

Jaap Valk, M. D., Ph. D.
Professor and Chairman,
Department of Neuroradiology
Academic Hospital Free University
Amsterdam
The Netherlands

x

Contents

Abbreviations

ADC	AIDS dementia complex
AIDP	Acute inflammatory demyelinating polyradiculoneuropathy
AIDS	Acquired immune deficiency syndrome
ARC	AIDS-related complex
ARDS	Adult respiratory distress syndrome
ARL	AIDS-related lymphoma
AZT	Zidovudine (azidothymidine)
BAL	Bronchoalveolar lavage
CDC	Centers for Disease Control
CIDP	Chronic inflammatory demyelinating polyradiculoneuropathy
CMV	Cytomegalovirus
CNS	Central nervous system
CSF	Cerebrospinal fluid
DHPG	Dihydroxyproproxymethyl-guanine
DSPN	Distal symmetric peripheral neuropathy
DTPA	Diethylene triamine penta acetic acid
ELISA	Enzyme-linked immunosorbent assay
Gd-DTPA	Gadolinium diethylene triamine penta acetic acid
GI	Gastrointestinal
gp	Glycoprotein
HBV	Hepatitis B virus
HIV	Human immunodeficiency virus
HPV	Human papillomavirus
HRCT	High-resolution computed tomography
HSV	Herpes simplex virus
HTLV-III	Human T-cell leukemia virus Type III
IBZM	3-Iodo-6-Methoxy-Benzamide
IVDU	Intravenous drug user
KS	Kaposi's sarcoma
LAV	Lymphandenopathy-associated virus
LIP	Lymphocytic interstitial pneumonitis
MAI	Mycobacterium avium – inter-cellulare
MM	Mononeuropathy multiplex
nef	negative regulatory factor
NHL	Non-Hodgkin's lymphoma
p	Protein
PA	Posterior – anterior
PCP	*Pneumocystis carinii* pneumonia
PET	Positron emission tomography
PML	Progressive multifocal leuko-encephalopathy
rCBF	Regional cerebral blood flow
rev	regulator of virion protein expression
SPECT	Single photon emission computed tomography
STD	Sexually transmitted disease
tat	transactivator protein
US	Ultrasonography
VZV	Varicella-zoster virus
WHO	World Health Organization

1 The Epidemiology of AIDS

P. J. E. Bindels, R. A. Coutinho

History

The acquired immune deficiency syndrome (AIDS) was first described in 1981 among young men in Los Angeles, San Francisco, and New York (1). These young men had in common that they were homosexual and had had a large number of sexual partners. Because of these findings AIDS was, at first, considered to be a disease restricted to the homosexual community. However, in the following years, AIDS was recognized among intravenous drug users (IVDUs) and Haitians (2, 3) as well. Shortly afterward, recipients of blood or blood products (4, 5), children of mothers at risk for AIDS (6), and heterosexual partners of AIDS patients (7) and Africans (8) were also found to suffer from AIDS. In the early years of the epidemic, several hypotheses about the cause of AIDS were formulated and then rejected, but it was soon clear that an agent transmittable via blood and via sexual contact had to be looked for. In 1983 a French group from the Pasteur Institute in Paris reported the isolation of a new retrovirus from the blood of a homosexual man with lymphadenopathy (9). They named the virus lymphadenopathy-associated virus (LAV). In 1984 American investigators from the National Institutes of Health also reported the isolation of a retrovirus, human T-cell Leukemia virus Type III (HTLV-III; 10, 11). Later, both viruses appeared to be similar and are now called the human immunodeficiency virus (HIV), considered to be the causative agent of AIDS.

Also in 1983, before the isolation of HIV, the Centers for Disease Control in Atlanta (CDC), developed a case definition for AIDS and described the diseases that were indicative of this specific immunodeficiency (e.g., a defect in cell-mediated immunity) and occurring in persons with no known cause for diminished resistance to disease. Diseases included in this first definition were *Pneumocystis carinii* pneumonia (PCP), *Candida* esophagitis, some other serious opportunistic infections and the aggressive form of Kaposi's sarcoma.

In 1985 a laboratory test became available to detect HIV antibodies. The availability of this test and the identification of the virus made it possible to start seroepidemiologic studies. It also made it necessary to revise the AIDS case definition that now included, for most cases, a positive HIV antibody test and a broader spectrum of diseases characteristically found in HIV antibody–positive persons (12). The World Health Organization (WHO) accepted this definition for worldwide use.

Since most African countries lack the adequate laboratory facilities needed to work with this case definition, the WHO developed a clinical definition of AIDS (13) to enable clinicians in these countries to diagnose the disease with maximum precision.

As the epidemic continued, more diseases and syndromes were described as occurring specifically in patients infected with HIV. As a result, the AIDS case definition developed by the CDC and WHO was revised again in 1987 (14). The most important diseases added in this last revision were extrapulmonary tuberculosis, HIV encephalopathy, HIV wasting syndrome, and the presumptive diagnosis of selected diseases (e.g., PCP). The 1987 revised case definition is now used as a guideline in most countries in which AIDS cases are diagnosed.

Transmission and the Natural History of Infection with HIV

Extensive studies have clarified the routes of transmission of HIV. The virus is transmitted through sexual contact with an infected person, through exposure to infected blood or blood products, and from an infected mother to her child (Table 1.1).

If a person is infected with HIV, acute clinical symptoms may occur. These acute symptoms have been described as a mononucleosis-like syndrome (Fig. 1.1), but a variety of other symptoms may also occur (flu, skin rash, arthralgia, etc.). These symptoms are not specific and not necessarily present and many persons notice no symptoms at all at the moment of acute infection.

Table 1.1   Routes of transmission of the human immunodeficiency virus (HIV)

Sexual	– Homosexual between men
	– Heterosexual from men to women and from women to men
Exposure to blood	– drug-user needle sharing
	– transfusion of blood, plasma, packed cells, platelet, and factor concentrates
	– occupational needle-prick injury
Perinatal	– prepartum, intrapartum, and possibly postpartum

HIV antibodies usually develop within 3 to 6 months after infection and can be detected by the available laboratory tests. Recently it has been suggested that, in sporadic cases, 6 or more months may elapse between infection and the development of HIV antibodies (15, 16).

Estimates of the time between infection and the development of AIDS (incubation time) vary from 6 months up to probably 15 years or more. Work regarding the distribution of incubation times has been done in cohort studies like the ones in San Francisco (San Francisco City Clinic Cohort Study and the San Francisco Mens' Health Study) and Amsterdam (J. C. M. Hendriks, unpublished data). Based on these studies, the *median* incubation time among adults in the Western world is estimated to be 8.5 to 11 years and the *mean* incubation time to vary from 9 to 12 years (17). The International Registry of Seroconverters, to which investigators from North America, Europe, and Australia have contributed data, has recently published similar results regarding AIDS incubation time among 1891 HIV seroconverters. The results of this study also show no differences in incubation times among homosexual men infected in different continents or in different years (18).

During the incubation period, an infected person is symptom-free and no clinical signs of an infection are present. However, transmission of the virus to uninfected persons is

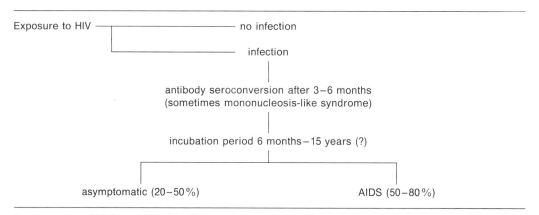

Fig. 1.1   Natural history of HIV infection

possible, and effective measures (e.g., safe-sex techniques, routine screening of blood donors) to prevent further spread of the virus are necessary.

It has been estimated recently (in a cohort study of homosexual and bisexual men) that 51% developed AIDS with 10 years of infection (19). However, there are investigators and clinicians who expect that this percentage will increase in the years to come and that eventually all infected persons will develop AIDS. The clinical symptoms leading to the diagnosis of AIDS will be discussed in chapter 3.

HIV is not transmitted through social contact, vaccines, or contact with insects or body fluids such as sweat or tears. Several epidemiologic studies and laboratory results have proved this. Unfortunately, it is not always believed, and myths about HIV and AIDS persist throughout the world. Assaults on the rights of infected persons and persons with AIDS are reported from many countries. This has, in some cases, led to an unjust social isolation of infected persons.

Routes of Transmission of HIV

Worldwide, three geographic patterns in the routes of transmission of HIV can be distinguished (20). In each pattern the main routes of transmission of HIV explain the distribution among the different risk groups in these countries.

Pattern 1 is typical of industrialized countries with large numbers of reported cases. In these countries most cases of AIDS are found among homosexual and bisexual men and intravenous drug users (through the sharing of needles). Most of them live in the urban areas of these countries, but the spread of HIV outside these areas is increasing. Only a small percentage of HIV-positive persons are infected through heterosexual contact. Their number is growing, especially in countries with high numbers of intravenous drug users or with many immigrants from pattern 2 areas. Due to the fact that most infected persons are male homosexuals or bisexuals,

relatively few women are seropositive, and therefore perinatal transmission is relatively rare. Transmission of the virus through blood transfusion or blood products has been extremely rare since tests to detect HIV antibodies became available (1985), and since the subsequent routine screening of donated blood was introduced and, in addition, the request that persons from the known risk groups refrain from donating blood.

The HIV seroprevalence in the overall population is estimated to be very low ($< 1\%$), but can be as high as 50% in certain risk groups in the urban areas (intravenous drug users and men with multiple male sex partners). Pattern 1 areas are the USA, Western Europe, and Australia.

In pattern 2 countries the majority of the cases occur among heterosexual persons. Men and women are equally affected and transmission from a mother to her child is a serious problem. Transmission of the virus through homosexual activity or the needle sharing of intravenous drug users is rare. Transmission of the virus through contaminated blood (products) is a considerable problem. Most pattern 2 countries are developing countries. This means that HIV antibody tests for routine screening are either not at hand or donor screening has not yet been implemented. Moreover, blood transfusion is an often-used therapy in these countries, and a shortage of injection needles as well as poor sterilization methods prior to the reuse of needles facilitates the spread of the virus. The high prevalence of (ulcerative) sexually transmitted diseases (STDs) in most of these countries is found to play a role in HIV transmission and can partly explain the large number of infected men and women (21, 22). HIV seroprevalence in the overall population is estimated at more than 1% and has reached 10% or more in the adult population of some capitals of these countries. Pattern 2 countries, sometimes called "AIDS endemic countries", are in the sub-Saharan regions of Africa (especially central and eastern Africa) and the Caribbean.

In most pattern 3 countries few AIDS cases have been reported up to now. The virus was probably introduced in these countries in the mid 1980s, and therefore the epidemic is in an early stage. Transmission occurs by way of all routes listed in Table 1.1. An increase in the number of AIDS cases in these countries could also be caused by a lack of sterile equipment and/or HIV test facilities (in cases of blood transfusion), as has been shown recently in Rumania where, up to and including September 1990, more than 900 children were diagnosed as having AIDS (23). Pattern 3 areas are the Eastern European countries, Asia, and the Pacific.

One should keep in mind that these patterns are not restricted to the above-mentioned countries. Interregional differences are seen within one pattern. The spread and routes of transmission of HIV are dynamic phenomena. An example for this is the recent rapid increase of AIDS cases seen in Brazil (more then 12000 cases by September 1990; 24). In this country, like in some other South American countries, a mixture of pattern 1 and 2 (homosexual and heterosexual transmission, as well as among intravenous drug users) is found.

AIDS Surveillance

Beginning with the diagnosis of the first AIDS patients, most countries in Western Europe, the USA, as well as some countries in Africa and other parts of the world introduced an AIDS surveillance system. The purpose of such epidemiologic surveillance is to keep authorities constantly informed about the course of the epidemic. The information obtained from this system is used to determine the needs of public health in the years to come and to assess the effectiveness of preventive programs (25). In most countries, AIDS surveillance is part of an already existing national surveillance system for infectious diseases. The WHO in Geneva coordinates the worldwide AIDS surveillance system and receives reports from the national surveillance systems and regional collaborating centers. AIDS cases reported to WHO are accepted if they meet either the CDC/WHO

definition or the WHO clinical definition. The WHO regularly publishes a global overview of the total number of reported AIDS patients in the different countries in their *Weekly Epidemiological Record*. The Centers for Disease Control (CDC) in Atlanta report on the trends in the epidemic in the USA, the country with the highest number of reported AIDS patients. Trends in the European AIDS epidemic are published quarterly by the WHO Collaborating Center on AIDS in Paris.

The completeness of AIDS case reporting and reporting delays are two items that have to be taken into account when evaluating or interpreting the figures provided by the above-mentioned organizations. The completeness of AIDS case reporting varies in different areas of the world. In Africa, for instance, it is known that AIDS case reporting is not carried out at all in several countries and has just recently started in others. Consequently, the reported numbers from Africa are an underestimation. In the USA many studies have evaluated the completeness of reporting (mainly through the comparison of death records and surveillance records). The results of these studies show considerable differences between areas. The completeness of reporting in the USA varied from 61% up to almost 100% (26). In Europe, the degree of underreporting varies between countries and over time. From 6 of the 12 European Community (EC) countries estimates varying from 0% to 20% are reported (27). A study carried out in Amsterdam in 1989 showed underreporting of 6% (28). The reporting delay, i.e., the time between diagnosis and reportage of an AIDS case, can vary between 1 month and more than 12 months and is therefore another factor to consider. Especially the most recent figures will be influenced by this reporting delay.

As mentioned above, the AIDS case definition was revised in 1985 and 1987. After the 1985 revision, the reported incidence of AIDS increased in the USA by only 3–4% (26). The 1987 revision had a much greater effect (an increase of more than 20%) on the number of reported cases. The possibility of a presumptive diagnosis, e.g., the inclusion of extra-pulmonary tuberculosis and the HIV wasting syndrome in the case definition, explains this increase. In Europe, the adoption of the 1987 revision of the AIDS case definition resulted in an estimated increase in the number of cases reported ranging from 0% to 28% for the different EC countries (27). It should be mentioned that some of these patients would have been reported with other AIDS criteria anyway at a later time and that the real impact of the revision is less than it appears.

In spite of these drawbacks, AIDS sur-veillance systems can provide a good im-pression of the influence and impact of the epidemic on today's world.

The Prevalence of AIDS and Its Trends

The presentation of recent cumulative num-bers of reported AIDS cases is limited by the fact that they will already be outdated tomor-row. Yet they are useful for describing the recent trends in the epidemic among the different risk groups.

By 31 December 1990 a total of 314 611 AIDS cases were reported to the World Health Organization in Geneva (29). Rough-ly half of the reported cases were diagnosed in the USA. Africa accounts for 81 019 cases (considerable underreporting suspected).

In this section the focus is on the trends and number of AIDS cases in Europe. This does not mean that the situation in other parts of the world will be left out. The Euro-pean situation is only used as a guideline and is more or less similar to the situation in the USA.

By 31 December 1990, AIDS surveillance in Europe (WHO Collaborating Center on AIDS, Paris) reported a total of 47 481 AIDS cases in 31 participating European countries (30). Since December 1989 the total number of reported cases in Europe had increased by 50.7% (15 984 new cases). In Figure 1.2 the cumulative number of AIDS cases for each European country is shown. Calculation of AIDS cases per million population for each country, based on 1989 population estimates, shows the highest cumulative incidence rate to be in Switzerland (242.9/million), France (234.1/million), and Spain (192.6/million). The incidence rate in the USA is 647.2 per million population (31). These estimates are cumulative incidence rates and therefore do not reflect the recent increase in the number of cases. During the last 3 months of 1990, France, Italy, and Spain were the countries with the greatest increases in the number of reported cases with 87–88, 50–51, and 34 newly reported cases per week, respectively.

Of the adult cases, 58.9% are between 25 and 40 years of age. Women are slightly younger than men at the time of diagnosis and represent roughly 14.5% of the total number of cases.

In Figure 1.3 the distribution of the cumu-lative number of AIDS cases among the different transmission categories is shown. In Europe, homosexual/bisexual men comprise the largest transmission group (44.1%), followed by intravenous drug users (31.2%), heterosexuals (8.3%), and recipients of blood or blood products (6.9%). Mother-to-child transmissions still represent less then 2% of the total number of cases.

If the distribution of AIDS cases is regard-ed by year of diagnosis, some interesting trends are seen (Fig. 1.4). In 1981 the first AIDS cases were reported in Europe, and, through the following years, the proportion of homosexual transmissions was the greatest. However, from 1985 onward, their proportion declined while the proportion of intravenous drug users increased. In 1984 they still represented less than 5% of the total number, but in 1989 their proportion was already 36%. For 1990, after correction for reporting delay, the absolute number of newly diagnosed AIDS cases among intra-venous drug users in that year will have been equal to or may have even exceeded the number among homosexual men. This rapid increase among intravenous drug users is mainly due to trends in countries like Italy and Spain. These countries have reported more AIDS cases in this group from the start of the epidemic (between 60 and 65% of the

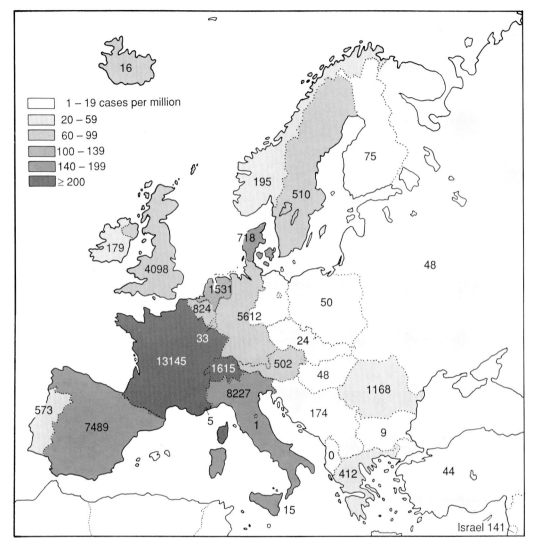

Fig. 1.**2**   Cumulative incidence rates per million population in Europe (WHO, 31 December 1990); n = 47 481

total number, compared to 5–15% for northern European countries).

The AIDS epidemic in a given population group is said to have three phases: an initial phase of rapidly increasing incidence (approximately exponential growth with constant doubling time), a second phase in which incidence increases progressively less rapidly (doubling times slowly increase), and a third phase in which the epidemic stabilizes or perhaps decreases.

Co-workers from the WHO Collaborating Center on AIDS (A. M. Downs, R. A. Ancelle, et al.) have frequently reported on the recent trends in Europe and for EC countries only (32). They applied different statistical models to routine AIDS surveillance data (1987–1989) to assess recent trends.

Their results for the EC countries (92% of AIDS cases in Europe) show that the estimated average doubling time, using the

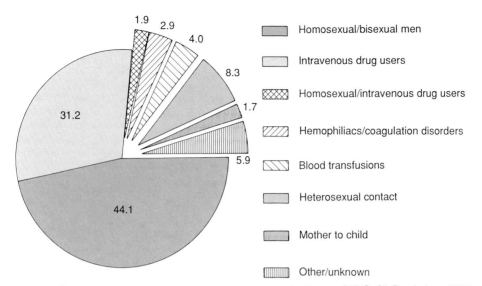

Fig. 1.3   Cumulative AIDS cases by transmission group in Europe (WHO, 31 December 1990); n = 47 481

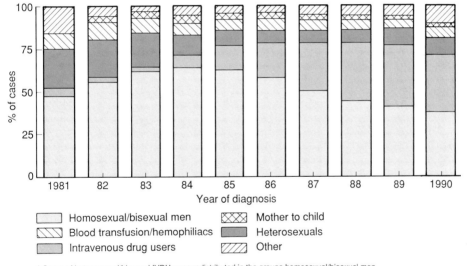

* Group of heterosexual/bisexual IVDUs was redistributed in the groups homosexual/bisexual men and intravenous drug users

Fig. 1.4   Transmission groups in Europe by year of diagnosis (WHO, 31 December 1990)

best-fitting model, for homosexual men has increased from 12 months in the period 1983– 1985 to 36 months in the most recent period. In the homosexual/bisexual transmission group, the rapidly increasing doubling times suggest a stabilizing or linear phase in the growth of the epidemic. This is particularly true for the countries in which homosexual males accounted for most cases from the beginning of the epidemic. For intravenous drug users the estimated doubling time is much shorter—16 months—which is reflected in the rapid increase of the number of cases in this group. Among intravenous drug users the doubling times are increasing, but not as rapidly as in the early phase of the epidemic in the homosexual group. The epidemic among intravenous drug users is still growing exponentially, although more stabilized growth is to be expected in this group as well. Despite an increase in doubling times from approximately 12 months (in the period July 1983 – June 1985) to a present estimate of 16 months among heterosexual persons, the epidemic in this group is still thought to be in an initial phase and further growth is likely to take place although a more linear growth pattern from the beginning is also a possibility.

In Europe 4.5% of the total number of cases occurs among children under 13 years of age. By 31 December 1990, 2120 children under 13 years of age at AIDS diagnosis were reported in Europe (Rumania accounted for 1094 of these cases!). In 38.5% of these cases, the child was infected perinatally by an HIV-seropositive mother (risk factor of mother: intravenous drug user, transfusion recipient, heterosexual contact and unknown risk factor). In the remaining 61.5% the child was infected through contaminated blood or blood products (29.5%) or the route of infection was unknown (32%, including patients infected by multiple injections). Besides Rumania, countries that contributed most to the number of pediatric cases are France, Italy, and Spain. These latter three countries are known because of their high proportion of intravenous drug users in the total number of cases. In contrast to other risk groups, a slight decline is estimate to have occurred, after adjustment for reporting delay, among children born to HIV-infected mothers between 1988 and 1990. This finding still has to be interpreted with caution. Nevertheless, this could be a result of testing women at risk for HIV infection and the counseling of these women regarding the consequences of such an infection for pregnancy (i.e., the resulting contraceptive measures and abortions).

When compared with the USA, no striking differences are seen. Through December 1990 homosexual/bisexual men formed the largest group (59%), followed by the group of intravenous drug users (22%). The percentage of IVDUs in the USA remained more or less stable over the years 1985–1987, but since 1988 the increase has continued. Males indulging in homosexual/bisexual contact and intravenous drug use represent 7% of cases, and heterosexual contact is thought to be the route of transmission in 5% of the cases (31). In the distribution of AIDS cases by race/ethnicity there is a trend that should be mentioned. An increasing number is diagnosed among minority groups (blacks and Hispanics). The high prevalence of intravenous drug abuse, socioeconomic factors and sexual behavior in these groups underlie this finding. In the years to come, this shift in emphasis toward minorities in the USA will probably continue and will demand extra (governmental) attention and preventive measures.

The distribution of AIDS cases in Africa is markedly different. More than 80% are acquired via heterosexual transmission and up to 10% of cases are due to transfusion of HIV-contaminated blood. Fewer than 1% are a result of intravenous drug abuse and approximately 5% are represented by homosexuals (34).

Prevalence of HIV

Although AIDS surveillance can provide us with much information about the trends in the number of AIDS patients, it is the epidemiology of HIV infection which provides a more complete and up-to-date view of what is to be expected in the near future. As pointed out above, the median and mean incubation times are estimated to vary between 8.5 and 12 years. This means that the number of AIDS patients diagnosed in one year reflects the situation of the HIV epidemic of several years back.

A reliable HIV surveillance is only present in a few countries and most information about the spread of HIV is obtained from seroprevalence studies among the known risk groups (mainly homosexual men and IVDUs) or other selected groups (visitors of STD clinics). Some of these studies will be discussed here in more detail.

In 1981, when AIDS was first recognized among homosexual men, substantial spread of the HIV had already occurred in this group. This became clear after seroepidemiologic studies of stored sera of homosexual men who were enrolled in hepatitis B studies at STD clinics in San Francisco between 1978 and 1980. A random sample was drawn from these sera and retrospective analysis revealed that HIV prevalence rose from 4.5% in 1978 to an estimated 44% by the end of 1981 (34). Similar prevalence data came from New York (35) and Los Angeles (36), two other epicenters of the AIDS epidemic. From these and other studies it appears that the introduction of HIV in the large urban centers of the USA took place in the mid-1970s. Studies outside the large urban centers have shown lower prevalence data for homosexual men, suggesting that in these areas fewer men were infected or they were infected at a later time.

In Western Europe the entry of HIV into the male homosexual community is thought to have happened some years later, at the end of the 1970s. Retrospective analysis of sera from homosexual men participating in a hepatitis B vaccine trial in Amsterdam revealed that 0.7% were infected with HIV in 1980 (37). Sera from homosexual men participating in a STD screening program in Stockholm showed that HIV was present in 2–6% in 1979 (38). Several cohort studies regarding the prevalence of HIV among homosexual men were carried out in the 1980s. These studies show a rising percentage of infected men in Europe, varying from 10 to 20% in the first years (39, 40) and 20 to 30% (41, 42) in the middle of the 1980s. In the late 1980s the first reports were published which showed a dramatic decrease in the incidence rates for new infection in cohort studies among homosexual men in Europe and North America. These incidence rates were estimated to be as high as 20% in 1982 and 1983 and dropped to 0.5–3% in 1987 and 1988 (43–45). An impressive change in sexual behavior among homosexual men influenced by targeted preventive campaigns (46, 47) is thought to be the reason for this decline. Subsequently it is possible that a more stable

seroprevalence will occur. However, most of these studies are carried out among relatively old homosexual men and one has to be cautious in extrapolating these results to younger groups of homosexual men.

In the second largest risk group for HIV infection, IVDUs, the virus was introduced in the USA (48) and Europe (49) in the mid- or late 1970s. It has been suggested that the sharing of needles between homosexual and heterosexual IVDUs has contributed to the introduction of HIV into this group (50). Next, the sharing of needles and syringes, caused by either a lack of sterile equipment, a sharing "tradition" in certain subcultures, or both facilitated a rapid spread of the virus. Early seroprevalence studies in the USA and Europe have confirmed these findings. In New York City, for example, seroprevalence rates went from 9% in 1978 to 60% in 1984 (48). A tragic example of rapid spread of HIV in a IVDU population has been documented recently in Thailand, where an increase in HIV prevalence from 0% in 1987 to 40% in 1988 was observed (51).

As is discussed above, there are considerable differences between north and south in the distribution of AIDS cases in Europe. HIV seroprevalences show the same pattern. In 1984–1985, high rates (44–53%) were already seen among IVDUs in Italy and Spain while much lower rates (1.5–6.4%) were observed in northern European countries. Recent cohort studies among IVDUs show more stable seroprevalence rates, as is seen among homosexual men. Whether this stabilization is also caused by behavioral change (safer use of injection equipment) is still questionable and might also be influenced by other factors (52).

In Europe and the USA, IVDUs play an important role in the transmission of HIV to non–drug-using heterosexuals (53). This occurs not only through sexual contact with their regular partner(s) but also through sexual contact with commercial partners (prostitution is a common way for IVDUs to get money to buy drugs). Sexual contact between bisexual men and heterosexual or bisexual women is another route for HIV into the heterosexual population. Heterosexual persons infected through contaminated blood products also contribute to this spread, but to a lesser extent.

There are few studies that report on seroprevalence rates among the general heterosexual population in Europe and the USA. Most of these studies are conducted among visitors of STD clinics and because of this selection, the results cannot be extrapolated to the general population. A recent study from as high a seroprevalence area as New York suggested that HIV infection among heterosexuals is still limited to sexual partners of intravenous drug users and of bisexual men and is low (1%) among persons outside all the known risk groups (54). In 1988 and 1989 a study was carried out in Amsterdam among pregnant women. The seroprevalence revealed was low (1988, 0.3% and 1989, 0.15%) and all seropositive women but one were members of the known risk groups or had had sexual contact with a person from a known risk group (including persons from pattern 2 countries; 55). Despite these low seroprevalence rates, caution is necessary because these results can be influenced by a relatively recent appearance of the virus in the heterosexual population. A recent rapid increase in cases attributed to heterosexual transmission in a country like Italy, where more than 60% of the reported AIDS cases occur among IVDUs, illustrates this.

HIV infection through contaminated blood has almost been eradicated since the routine HIV antibody screening of blood (products) started in most Western countries in 1985. Nevertheless, persons donating blood while in the "window-phase" (time between infection and the presence of HIV antibodies) can still infect recipients.

A discussion of the situation in Africa will conclude this section. Heterosexual transmission is the major route and high HIV seroprevalences in the general population are documented in some African countries with dramatic figures: 20% among urban adults in Rwanda (1987; 56); a seroprevalence among prostitutes in Kampala of 90% (33). At the present time, HIV infection and AIDS occur predominantly in urban centers and to a lesser extent in rural areas, where most Africans (roughly 80%) live (33, 57). Unfortunately, the epidemic has not yet stabilized, and the impact of the HIV epidemic on the social and economic development of these highly endemic African countries is already tremendous and will become even worse in the years to come.

Prediction of AIDS Cases

To develop public health care policies and to evaluate the preventive measures applied, predictions of the course of the AIDS epidemic are necessary. The first projections were based on extrapolation of the observed incidence of AIDS cases and predicted an exponential growth of the number of cases in the early years. This led to an overestimation of the expected number of cases. By now, many complicated mathematical models have been developed in which a variety of factors can be incorporated. This brings about another problem: even in short-term prediction, which is common nowadays, the different models may produce significantly different results. Therefore, all predictions should be interpreted with extreme caution, and the assumptions and limitations of each mathematical model should be taken into account.

For the European Community countries, a short-term prediction with the above-mentioned reservations, for the end of 1991 lies somewhere between cumulative 60000 and 78000 cases, of which 24000–30000 projected cases are among homosexual and bisexual men, 23000–33000 are among IVDUs, and 6000–8000 are in the heterosexual transmission group (32).

References

1. Centers for Disease Control. Pneumocystis pneumonia, Los Angeles. MMWR 1981;30:250–2.
2. Centers for Disease Control. Update on Kaposi's sarcoma and opportunistic infections in previously healthy persons: United States. MMWR 1982;31:294–301.

3. Centers for Disease Control. Opportunistic infections and Kaposi's sarcoma among Haitians in the United States. MMWR 1982; 31:353–61.

4. Centers for Disease Control. Update on acquired immune deficiency syndrome (AIDS) among patients with hemophilia A. MMWR 1982; 31:644–52.

5. Centers for Disease Control. Possible transfusion-associated acquired immune deficiency syndrome (AIDS): California. MMWR 1982; 31:652–4.

6. Centers for Disease Control. Unexplained immunodeficiency and opportunistic infections in infants: New York, New Jersey, California. MMWR 1982; 31:665–8.

7. Centers for Disease Control. Immunodeficiency among female sexual partners of males with acquired immune deficiency snydrom (AIDS): New York. MMWR 1983; 31:697–8.

8. Clumeck N, Mascart-Lemone F, de Manbeuge J, et al. Acquired immune deficiency syndrome in black Africans. Lancet 1983; 1:642.

9. Barré-Sinoussi F, Cherman JC, Raij F, et al. Isolation of a T-lymphotropic retrovirus from a patient at risk for acquired immunodeficiency syndrome. Science 1983; 220:868–70.

10. Popovic M, Sarngadharan MG, Read E, Gallo RC. Detection, isolation and continuous production of cytopathic retrovirus (HTLV-III) from patients with AIDS and at risk for AIDS. Science 1984; 224:500–503.

11. Levy JA, Hoffman AD, Kramer SM, et al. Isolation of lymphocytopathic retroviruses from San Francisco patients with AIDS. Science 1984; 225:840–2.

12. Centers for Disease Control. Revision of the case definition of acquired immuno deficiency syndrome for national reporting. MMWR 1985; 34:373–5.

13. World Health Organisation. Acquired immune deficiency syndrome (AIDS): WHO/CDC case definition for AIDS. Wkly Epidemiol Rec 1986; 61:69–73.

14. Centers for Disease Control. Revision of the CDC surveillance case definition for acquired immune deficiency syndrome. MMWR 1987; 36 (suppl. 1 S)

15. Horsburgh CR, Jason J, Longini IM, et al. Duration of human immunodeficiency virus infection before detection of antibody. Lancet 1989; 11:637–9.

16. Imagawa DT, Lee MH, Wolinsky JM, et al. Human immunodeficiency virus Type 1 infection in homosexual men who remain seronegative for prolonged period. N Engl J med 1989; 320:1458–62.

17. Lemp GF, Payne SF, Rutherford GW, et al. Projections of AIDS morbidity and mortality in San Francisco. JAMA 1990; 263:1497–1501.

18. Biggar JR and The International Registry of Seroconverters. AIDS incubation in 1891 HIV seroconverters from different exposure groups. AIDS 1990; 4:1059–1066.

19. Lifson AR, Hessol N, Rutherford G, et al. Natural history of HIV-infection in a cohort of homosexual and bisexual men: clinical and immunologic outcome. From: Sixth international conference on AIDS, San Francisco, USA, 1990, vol 1 (Abstract Th. C. 33).

20. Centers for Disease Control. Update: acquired immune deficiency syndrome (AIDS) worldwide. MMWR 1988; 37:286–95.

21. Pepin J, Plummer FA, Brunham RC, et al. The interaction of HIV-infection and other sexually transmited diseases: an opportunity for intervention. AIDS 1989; 3:3–10.

22. Berkley SF, Widy-Wirsky R, Okware SI, et al. Risk factors associated with HIV-infection in Uganda. J Infect Dis 1989; 160:22–30.

23. WHO Collaborating Center on AIDS, Paris. AIDS surveillance in Europe: quarterly report no. 27, September 1990.

24. World Health Organization. Weekly epidemiological record. Geneva, 11 January 1991.

25. Centers for Disease Control. Guidelines for evaluating surveillance systems. MMWR 1988; 37 (suppl. S-5).

26. Centers for Disease Control. AIDS and human immunodeficiency virus infection in the United States: 1988 update. MMWR 1989; 38 (suppl. S-4).

27. WHO Collaborating Center on AIDS, Paris. AIDS surveillance in Europe: quarterly report no. 23, September 1989.

28. Bindels PJE, Jong JTL, Poos HJJ, et al. The epidemiology of AIDS in Amsterdam, 1982–1988. Ned Tijdschr Geneeskd 1990; 134:390–4.

29. World Health Organization. Weekly epidemiological record. Geneva, 11 January 1991.

30. WHO Collaborating Center on AIDS, Paris. AIDS surveillance in Europe: quarterly report no. 28, December 1990.

31. Centers for Disease Control. HIV/AIDS surveillance report, January 1991; 1–22.

32. Downs AM, Ancella-Park RA, Brunet J-B. Surveillance of AIDS in the European community: recent trends and predictions to 1991. AIDS 1990; 4:1117–24.

33. N'Gali B, Bertozzi S, Ryder RW, Obstacles to the optimal management of HIV-infections/AIDS in Africa. J Acquired Immune Deficiency Syndromes 1990; 3:403–7.

34. Jaffe HW, Darrow WW, Eckenberg DF, et al. The acquired immunodeficiency syndrome in cohort of homosexual men: a six-year follow-up study. Ann Intern Med 1985; 97:362–6.

35. Stevens CE, Taylor PE, Zang EA, et al. Human T-cell lymphotropic virus Type III infection in a cohort of homosexual men in New York City. JAMA 1986; 255:2167–72.

36. De Cock KM, Niland JC, Hsiao-Ping LU, et al. Experience with human immunodeficiency virus infection in patients with hepatitis B virus and hepatitis B delta virus infections in Los Angeles, 1977–1985. Am J Epidemiol 1988; 127:1250–60.

37. Coutinho RA, Krone WJA, Smit J, et al. The introduction of LAV/HTLV III into the male homosexual community in Amsterdam. Genitourin Med 1986; 62:38–43.

38. Von Krosh G, Brostrom C, Hermanson J, et al. The introduction of HIV during 1979–1980 in a sexually active homosexual population of Stockholm. Scand J Infect Dis 1987; 29:285–8.

39. Melbye M, Biggar RJ, Ebbesen P, et al. Seroepidemiology of HTLV-III antibody in Danish homosexual men: prevalence, transmission, and disease outcome. Br Med J 1984; 289:537–45.

40. Weber JN, Wadsworth J, Rogers LA, et al. Three-year prospective study of LAV/HTLV in infection in homosexual men. Lancet 1986; 1179–82.

41. Ross MGR, MacDonald Burns D, Grundy JE, et al. Infection with human immunodeficiency virus (HIV) and cytomegalovirus in a London health district, 1980–4. Genitourin Med 1987; 63:28–31.

42. Blaser J, Lüthy R, Rietiker S, Ledergerber B, Täuber MG. Prevalence of HIV antibodies in groups at risk in Zurich, Switzerland. Klin Wochenschr 1987; 65:245–6.

43. Hessol NA, O'Malley P, Lifson A, et al. Incidence and prevalence of HIV infection among homosexual and bisexual men, 1978–1988. Fifth international conference on AIDS. Montreal, June 1989 (abstract M.A.O. 27).

44. Winkelstein W, Samuel M, Padian NS, et al. San Francisco men's health study III: reduction in human immunodeficiency virus transmission among homosexual/bisexual men, 1982–1986. Am J Public Health 1987; 77:685–9.

45. Griensven GJP van, de Vroome EMM, Goudsmit J, Coutinho RA. Changes in sexual behaviour and the fall in incidence of HIV infection among homosexual men. Br Med J 1989; 298:218.

46. Griensven GJP van, de Vroome EMM, Goudsmit J, Coutinho RA. Changes in sexual behaviour connected to strong decline in HIV incidence among homosexual men. Fifth international conference on AIDS, Montreal, June 1989 (abstract T.A.P. 20).

47. Coutinho RA, van Griensven GJP, Moss A. Effects of preventive efforts among homosexual men. AIDS 1989; 3:S53–S56.

48. Des Jarlais DC, Friedman SR, Novick DM, et al. HIV-1 infection among intravenous drug users in Manhattan, New York City, from 1977 through 1987. JAMA 1989; 261:1008–12.

49. Titti F, Lazzarin A, Costiglida P, et al. Human immunodeficiency virus (HIV) seropositivity in intravenous (IV) drug abusers in three cities of Italy: possible natural history of HIV infection in IV drug addicts in Italy. J Med Virol 1987; 23:241–8.

50. Battjes RJ, Dickens RW, Amstel Z. Introduction of HIV infection among intravenous drug users in low-prevalence areas. J Acquired Immune Deficiency Syndromes 1989; 2:533–9.

51. Coutinho RA, Epidemiology and prevention of AIDS among intravenous drug users. J Acquired Immune Deficiency Syndromes 1990; 4:413–16.

52. Hartgers C. AIDS and drugs. AIDS Care 1989; 2:206–11.

53. Hoek JAR van den, van Haastrecht HJA, Coutinho RA. Heterosexual behaviour of intravenous drugusers in Amsterdam. AIDS 1990; 4:449–53.

54. Chiasson MA, Stoneburner RL, Lifson AR, et al. Risk factors for human immunodeficiency virus type I (HIV-1) infection in patients at a sexually transmitted disease clinic in New York City. Am J Epidemiol 1990; 131:208–20.

55. Coutinho RA, Boer K, Schutte MF, et al. Prevalence of HIV among pregnant women in and around Amsterdam in 1989. Ned Tijdschr Geneeskd 1990; 134:1264–6.

56. Rwandan HIV Prevalence Study Group. Nationwide community-based serological survey of HIV-1 and other human retrovirus infections in a central African country. Lancet 1989; 1: 947–9.

57. Piot P, Laga M, Ryder R, et al. The global epidemiology of HIV infection: continuity, heterogeneity, and change. J Acquired Immune Deficiency Syndromes 1990; 4:403–11.

2 The Pathology of AIDS

J. G. van den Tweel, M. E. I. Schipper

The diagnosis AIDS will be established in HIV-positive patients if there is mention of the following CDC criteria:

1. opportunistic infections,
2. Kaposi's sarcoma,
3. malignant lymphoma with a high degree of malignancy,
4. AIDS encephalopathy,
5. lymphocytic interstitial pneumonitis (LIP) in HIV-positive children, or
6. HIV wasting syndrome.

Opportunistic Infections

Opportunistic infections are mainly found in three organ systems: the respiratory tract, the digestive tract, and the central nervous system. The most important infections in these tracts are described here briefly.

Respiratory Tract

Pneumocystis carinii

Pneumocystis carinii pneumonia is a frequently occurring infection of the lung which is observed in most AIDS patients. It presents as bilateral interstitial pneumonitis with little other clinical symptomatology. The diagnosis is established by demonstrating *Pneumocystis carinii* organisms in bronchial lavages or in lung biopsies. The combination of bronchial lavage and peripheral biopsy produces a reliable diagnosis in more than 90% of cases. *Pneumocystis carinii* is a commensal protozoon in the pulmonary tissue of man and mammals. The parasite varies from 3 to 5 μm in diameter and presents in the form of a trophozoite or oocyte in the alveolar exudate. The parasites can be visualized with the help of Giemsa, toluidine blue, or Grocott staining. In routine H and E staining, the alveoli are filled with a strongly eosinophilic, cloudy exudate. The adjacent pulmonary tissue demonstrates strikingly few signs of infection.

Cytomegalovirus

Cytomegalovirus infections usually occur at a later stage of AIDS, and if not recognized, have a very poor prognosis. If pneumonia is recognized, the prognosis is favorable. The quickest diagnosis can be achieved by performing a cytologic assessment of a bronchoalveolar lavage (BAL), complemented by immunohistochemical analysis of the infiltrate using monoclonal antibodies directed at CMV. A positive cytology (whether based on immunocyto-chemistry or not) is almost always specific for CMV pneumonia. The virus is present in endothelial cells but also in the pneumocytes. It manifests itself as eosinophilic inclusion bodies in the nucleus or cell cytoplasm (Figs. 2.**1**, 2.**2**).

Cryptococcus neoformans

Cryptococcal pneumonia strongly resembles a *Pneumocystis carinii* pneumonia or a

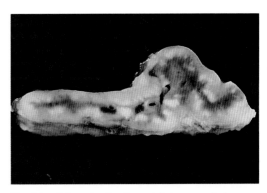

Fig. 2.**1** Adrenal gland containing small hemorrhages in the medulla and white spotted foci of necrosis caused by CMV infection

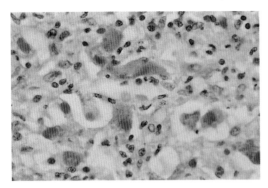

Fig. 2.2 Microscopic image of adrenal gland infected with CMV. The large dark purple cells reveal viral inclusions

cytomegalovirus infection. The cryptococci can easily be demonstrated in a bronchial lavage or lung biopsy using a PAS or Grocott stain. The cryptococcal yeasts are 4 to 7 μm in diameter and form short, plump spores. The transparent capsule around the yeast (*Cryptococcus neoformans capsulatum*) is characteristic. This is composed of mucopolysaccharides which are also responsible for the staining with PAS and the Grocott stain. Organisms are situated mainly extracellularly or intracellularly in macrophages. This infection too is accompanied by an amazingly slight response.

Mycobacterium avium–intracellulare

Infection with MAI usually appears in the form of a disseminated mycobacterial infection (Fig. 2.3). MAI is present in histiocytes and does not cause granulomatous inflammation, as is the case with tuberculosis (Fig. 2.5). The microorganisms can be revealed with a routine Ziehl–Neelsen stain.

Digestive Tract

The digestive tract is often affected early in the disease by opportunistic infections. These abnormalities may be present anywhere between the mouth and the anus. Chronic diarrhea and progressive weight loss are the most important clinical symptoms of this type of infection.

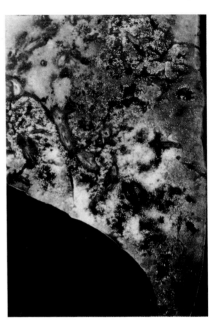

Fig. 2.3 Lung demonstrating dark red foci of a Kaposi sarcoma, mainly localized around blood vessels. The white areas are due to infection with *Mycobacterium avium – intracellulare*

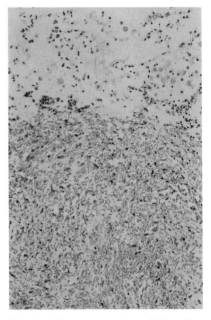

Fig. 2.4 Microscopic view of Kaposi's sarcoma in the lungs. The vascular spaces are filled with erythrocytes. Pre-existent alveolar lung tissue is also present

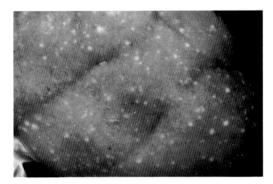

Fig. 2.**5** Kidney surface showing multiple small foci of tuberculosis

Protozoa

Gastrointestinal infections with protozoa mainly involve *Cryptosporidium*, *Microsporidium* and *Isospora belli*.

None of these three pathogens is a frequent cause of a disease entity. *Cryptosporidium* occurs in both the small and large intestines, while *Microsporidium* and *Isospora belli* are mainly found in the epithelium of the small intestine. The microsporidians, which have a diameter of less than 1 μm, are very difficult to diagnose. Electron microscopy is essential if the diagnosis is to be established with any certainty. *Cryptosporidium* protozoa are 2–6 μm long, while *Isospora belli* oocysts measure 15 to 30 μm.

Cytomegalovirus

A cytomegalovirus infection of the digestive tract is a relatively frequently occurring complication of AIDS (Fig. 2.**6**). Just as in the respiratory tract, the virus particles are mainly found in the nuclei and the cytoplasm of the vascular endothelium. It is not, however, unusual for the epithelium to be affected. In the case of the CMV, the entire gastrointestinal canal can be infected (Fig. 2.**7**).

Mycobacterium avium–intracellulare

MAI infection of the gastrointestinal tract is not usually diagnosed until later in the course

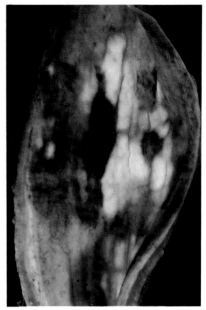

Fig. 2.**6** Esophagus containing only a few (white) areas with normal squamous cell epithelium. The dark red central focus is a Kaposi sarcoma. The other red-injected mucous membrane demonstrates a CMV infection

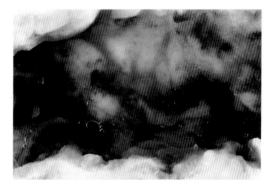

Fig. 2.**7** Large intestine with an ulcerative inflammation as a result of CMV infection

of the disease. On the whole, the infection is not fatal. The microorganisms are found in macrophages which are localized in the stroma of the villi and in the lamina propria of the mucosa (Figs. 2.**8**, 2.**9**).

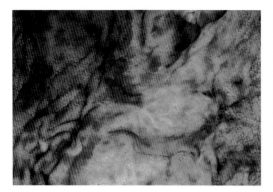

Fig. 2.**8**   Gastric mucosa containing diffuse, multiple, small, white foci of *Mycobacterium avium*

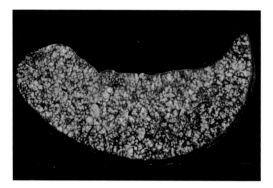

Fig. 2.**9**   Spleen extensively infected with *Mycobacterium avium*

Cryptococci

In a disseminated cryptococcosis, the fungus can also be located in the digestive tract. This infection is accompanied by the production of a considerable amount of mucus which results in destruction of the tissue in the midst of which the microorganisms are stored. Often the only observed reaction is the formation in the cytoplasm of multinucleate giant cells with cryptococci.

Candida albicans

Many HIV-positive patients develop *Candida* infections of the mouth and the esophagus. A thick coating of the normal mucous membrane is a characteristic feature (Fig. 2.**10**). The fungal filaments can be visualized using

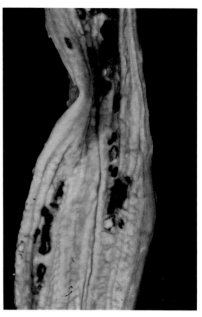

Fig. 2.**10**   Esophagus with a widespread *Candida* infection and with black, sharply defined erosions due to reflux

an H and E stain, but a PAS or Grocott stain facilitates the diagnosis in cases of doubt. The yeast cells are 3 to 4 μm long and demonstrate characteristic budding, with the formation of pseudohyphae which infiltrate the epithelium. *Candida albicans* can cause enteritis, but this is a relatively rare occurrence.

Central Nervous System

Although the number of patients who present with neurologic symptoms fluctuates around 30%, autopsy reveals that more than 80% of the patients have cerebral abnormalities. These abnormalities are largely caused by *Toxoplasma gondii* infections. Fungal infections are less frequent. On the other hand, viral infections, in particular direct effects of HIV, are fairly frequent.

Toxoplasma gondii

Intracerebral infection with the protozoon *Toxoplasma gondii* is a frequent occurrence in

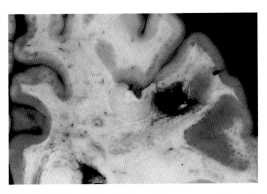

Fig. 2.**11**   Frontal brain lobe with an area of sharply delineated caseating necrosis. Lateral of this, one can see a hemorrhage in the white matter of the gyrus frontalis inferior. This sharply delineated process is caused by *Toxoplasma gondii*

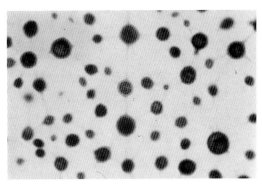

Fig. 2.**12**   Cerebrospinal fluid containing a cryptococcus infection (PAS stain)

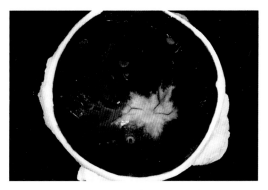

Fig. 2.**13**   Irregular, white (cotton wool) spot due to CMV infection of the retina

AIDS patients. The illness manifests as an acute, subacute, or chronic necrotizing inflammation of the cerebrum with the development of neurologic signs, fever, and sometimes a lowered level of consciousness. The IgG toxoplasmosis titers are often raised, which indicates that the cerebral infection is probably a reactivation of a previous infection. In cerebro, necrotic foci (Fig. 2.**11**) are found in which the characteristic 2–6 µm tachyzoites and/or cysts can be demonstrated. Reactive changes can be seen at the edge of the foci, with little inflammatory infiltrate and sometimes a multinucleate giant cell.

Cryptococci and Candida albicans

Both fungal infections cause clinical signs which are like those of toxoplasmosis (Fig. 2.**12**). These have already been described in this chapter.

Papovavirus

The JC-virus, a virus of the papova group, causes a progressive multifocal leukoencephalopathy. This virus infection causes the progressive multifocal demyelinization which results in this clinical picture. The virus can also be demonstrated in the oligodendrocytes and astrocytes. The infection of the oligodendroglia cells produces reactive, swollen, bizarre astrocytes. This picture is histologically characteristic of a papovavirus infection.

Cytomegalovirus

The cytomegalovirus infection often expresses itself in the first instance as a retinitis (Fig. 2.**13**). In cerebro, small foci of inflammation can be found in both gray and white matter (Fig. 2.**14**). The peripheral nervous system is hardly ever affected by this virus.

HIV

In cerebro, the HIV causes progressive encephalopathy accompanied by dementia. In

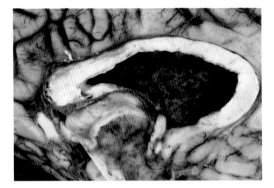

Fig. 2.**14** Sagittal section through the brain. The ventricle wall contains a hemorrhagic lesion due to a cytomegalovirus infection

the gray and white matter, the morphologic substrate consists of microglial nodules, together with signs of diffuse, slight demyelination as well as reactive gliosis. Macrophages are found perivascularly. Since the introduction of routine AZT therapy, AIDS encephalopathy appears relatively seldom.

Kaposi's Sarcoma

Until the 1980s, Kaposi's sarcoma was a relatively rare tumor. It was first described a century ago in men and women between 50 and 70 years of age. It was not until it appeared in AIDS patients that Kaposi's sarcoma became a frequently occurring tumor in the Western world. Macroscopically, early Kaposi's sarcoma is characterized by purple nodules. Microscopic examination reveals irregularly dilated vascular spaces coated with swollen endothelial cells. At a later stage, the endothelium may demonstrate some nuclear polymorphism and mitoses may appear here and there. Extravasation of erythrocytes and accompanying deposits of iron pigment complete the picture. An important diagnostic criterion in the diagnosis of this disease process is that there are small vascular spaces which are formed by a single endothelial cell.

This process does not only occur in the skin; all organ systems can be affected

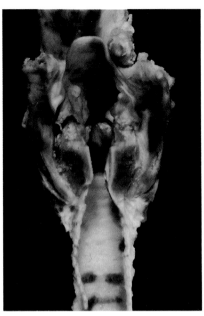

Fig. 2.**15** Pharynx and trachea; various sites show widespread Kaposi's sarcoma

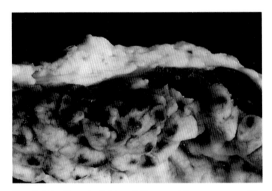

Fig. 2.**16** Rough folds of the gastric mucosa with small, red Kaposi's sarcoma foci at various sites

(Fig. 2.**4**). In particular, the digestive tract is a frequent site of this tumor (Figs. 2.**15**–**18**).

Malignant Lymphoma

The malignant lymphomas which are found in AIDS patients are nearly always B-cell lymphomas. T-cell lymphomas are exceptions. The degree of malignancy of these tumors is always intermediate or high. This implies that the centroblastic lymphomas,

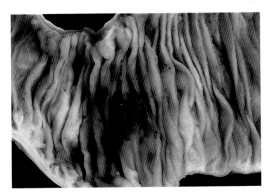

Fig. 2.**17** Small intestine (jejunum) with an area containing a Kaposi sarcoma at its center

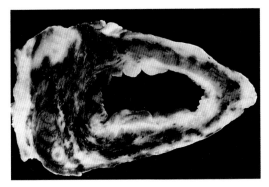

Fig. 2.**18** Transverse section of the myocardium showing widespread Kaposi's sarcoma

lymphoblastic lymphomas, and immunoblastic lymphomas compose the majority of malignant lymphomas in AIDS patients. Studies indicate that the Epstein–Barr virus can often be demonstrated in these tumors. Not only is the incidence of malignant lymphomas in AIDS patients considerably increased, but in particular the occurrence of cerebral lymphomas is often observed in AIDS patients. In these cases, the lymphoma is often confined to the cerebrum.

AIDS Encephalopathy

AIDS encephalopathy is a syndrome which is caused by the human immunodeficiency virus. It has already been described in the section on viral infections of the central nervous system.

Lymphocytic Interstitial Pneumonitis

LIP is a syndrome in which dense, lymphoid infiltrates occur in the alveolar septa of the lung. This picture is sometimes difficult to distinguish from a malignant lymphoma; if it occurs in HIV-positive children, it gives rise to the diagnosis of AIDS. In adults, however, the appearance of this syndrome is not a criterion for AIDS diagnosis.

HIV wasting syndrome

This syndrome has no pathological substrate and will not be discussed in this chapter.

References

Alonzo R, Heiman-Patterson T, Mancall EL. Cerebral toxoplasmosis in acquired immune deficiency syndrome. Arch Neurol 1984; 41:321.

CDC. Revision of the CDC surveillance case definition for acquired immunodeficiency syndrome. MMWR 1987; 35 (suppl. no. 15).

CDC. Classification system for human immunodeficiency virus (HIV) infection in children under 13 years of age. MMWR 1987; 36:225–30, 235.

Cohen RJ, Sameszuk MK, Busch, et al. Occult infections with mycobacterium avium–intracellulare in bone marrow biopsy specimens from patients with AIDS. N Engl J Med 1983; 308:1475.

Epstein CG, et al. Neurologic manifestations of human immunodeficiency virus infection in children. Pediatrics 1986; 78:678.

Guarda LA, Luna MA, Smith JL, et al. Acquired immune deficiency syndrome: postmortem findings. Am J Clin Pathol 1984; 81:549.

Hinnant KL et al. Cytomegalovirus infection of the alimentary tract: a clinicopathological correlation. Am J Gastroenterol 1986; 81:944.

Ioachim HL. Pathology of AIDS. London: Gower Medical, 1989.

Lander I. The lymphadenopathy of human immunodeficiency virus infection. Histopathology 1986; 10:1203.

Lefkowith JH, Krumholz S, Feng-Chen K, et al. Cryptosporidiosis of the human small intestine: a light and electron microscopic study. Hum Pathol 1984; 15:476.

Marray JF, Felton CP, Garay SM, et al. Pulmonary complications of the acquired immunodeficiency syndrome. N Engl J Med 1984; 310:1682.

Morris JC, Rosen MJ, Marchevsky A, et al. Lymphocytic interstitial pneumonia in patients at risk for the acquired immune deficiency syndrome. Chest 91; 1987; 1:63.

3 Clinical Diagnostics in AIDS

S. A. Danner

The diagnosis of AIDS is a clinical one. Laboratory investigation is essential (HIV antibodies), but the diagnosis can only be established if, in addition to HIV seropositivity, one or more well-described clinical syndromes are present.

The original diagnosis of AIDS, as employed for epidemiologic research, was adjusted several times as more became known about the various syndromes which can cause immunosuppression as seen in HIV infection.

The practicing clinician will not, however, be satisfied with the diagnosis: AIDS or no AIDS. If he or she is to give as accurate a prognosis as possible in each individual case and to instigate optimal therapy, he or she has to know how far the disease process of the HIV infection, of which the last phase is represented by AIDS, has advanced in the patient.

For this reason, a few clinical classification systems have been devised, of which the CDC (Centers for Disease Control, Atlanta, USA) system is the most used. This system consists of 4 major groups which are mutually exclusive; a patient with an HIV infection will only belong to one of these classes. Class I is the acute HIV infection. Class II is the asymptomatic HIV infection. Class III is composed of patients with persistent generalized lymphadenopathy. Finally, class IV consists of patients with symptoms. This last class is subdivided into 5 groups, and a patient can belong to more than one subgroup. Subgroup IV-A includes the most severe constitutional symptoms (continuing diarrhea and fever e.c.i. (*e causa ignota*), severe weight loss, severe tiredness, and a feeling of being unwell), IV-B a number of neurologic syndromes as a result of the HIV infection, IV-C the infections, IV-D the malignancies, and IV-E a remainder consisting of various disorders which in themselves have something to do with the HIV infection but which cannot be classified (e.g., autoimmune thrombocytopenia). Disorders in some groups do lead to a diagnosis of AIDS.

The acute HIV infection, CDC class I, occurs slightly more frequently than originally assumed, but the signs are not usually recognized. One is dealing with a mononucleosis-type syndrome with fever, swelling of the lymph glands, sometimes skin rash, problems with the joints, sometimes an aseptic meningitis, and sometimes ulcers in the digestive tract, lasting on the whole 3–5 weeks. If a patient presenting with such a picture belongs to one of the risk groups for HIV infection, one should certainly consider this and discuss how to determine HIV serology. HIV-p24 antigen first becomes detectable in the peripheral blood, often only for a short time (a few days, sometimes a few weeks). If the antigenicity starts to fall, HIV antibodies usually appear in the blood, and the patient is determined to be seropositive when the blood is screened. Sporadically there may be a short period in which the antigen has already disappeared from the blood while the antibodies are not yet demonstrable. In this case there is a danger of missing the diagnosis, even when it is suspected clinically. One should then carry out a follow-up study on the patient.

The asymptomatic HIV infection, class II, can roughly be divided into a period in which the number of CD4+ cells (T-helper lymphocytes) is normal, and a period in which it is too low. The first period can last a considerable length of time and covers the largest part of the incubation time of this disease. If the number begins to fall, it does not usually take long (6–9 months) for the patient to develop symptoms, whereby he or she then ends up in class IV.

CDC class III also consists of people who actually do not have any complaints but one, namely a generalized lymph gland swelling, which is the consequence of the HIV infection and not some opportunistic infection. These individuals in fact behave in the same way as those in class II. The lymph gland tumor can exist for months or years without exerting any clear influence on the prognosis. If one ends up in class IV-A (serious constitutional symptoms), then it is usually not very long before some complication or other arises on the basis of which the diagnosis AIDS is established.

The classification as outlined above is important both for the prognosis and for the therapeutic approach. Recently, an agreement has been reached to treat patients, even if they are symptom-free, with primary prophylaxis against the occurrence of a *Pneumocystis carinii* pneumonia as soon as the number of CD4+ cells is less than 200/mm^3. Furthermore, prophylactic treatment of class II individuals who have less than 500/mm^3 CD4+ cells with an anti-HIV substance—zidovudine, or AZT—is under consideration.

The clinical diagnostics of the various AIDS complications is strongly dependent on the organ involved. In general, four organ systems are affected: the bronchial/respiratory organs, the gastrointestinal canal, the central nervous system (including the eyes), and the skin. It is beyond the scope of this chapter to discuss the various disorders in detail, but the following should be pointed out:

A symptomatic patient infected with HIV regularly develops new symptoms. Each symptom can be indicative of many disorders. The textbooks state which investigation is indicated for which symptom for the purpose of establishing a diagnosis. However, the investigation is usually invasive. Sooner or later, patients will refuse to undergo any more investigations. Not because they think they know better, nor because they want to die, but simply because they have had enough and have the feeling that they cannot take any more. When dealing with HIV infection and AIDS, it is advisable—more so than with some other diseases—to continually weigh up the expected pros and cons of each investigation.

4 AIDS: a Retrovirus Infection in Humans

C. A. B. Boucher, J. Goudsmit

The aquired immune deficiency syndrome (AIDS) is characterized by the appearance of opportunistic infections and tumors. Generally, AIDS does not emerge until years after the infection with the human immunodeficiency virus (HIV) has actually occurred. This chapter discusses the course and diagnostics of the infection, the structure and replication of HIV, and the pathogenesis and treatment of HIV infections.

The Course of an HIV Infection

The case history of a 58-year-old woman illustrates the full extent of the course of an HIV infection (Fig. 4.1). In January, 1985, she was admitted to the hospital with a serious form of the Guillain–Barré syndrome. The decision was made to treat her with plasmapheresis, and for 2 weeks her plasma was replaced by a total of 16 L of plasma derived from 82 different plasma donors. Two and a half years after the plasmapheresis, a Kaposi sarcoma and a *Candida* esophagitis were diagnosed. Also at that time, HIV antibodies could be demonstrated. In her case, the plasmapheresis procedure was the most probable source of HIV infection.

Retrospective analysis of the plasma samples with which she had been treated revealed that one plasma sample contained HIV antibodies. On the basis of stored serum samples from the patient, the development of serologic parameters could be investigated.

Using the HIV antigen test, proteins originating from the core of the virus can be detected in serum. Two weeks after the infection, HIV antigen was found in her serum for a period of 1 week. The presence of these viral core proteins in her serum indicates that viral replication was occurring in the patient's cells. This was followed by the detection of HIV antibodies in her serum.

Some of the HIV antibodies are directed against the viral core and these antibodies can bind with the viral core proteins and form

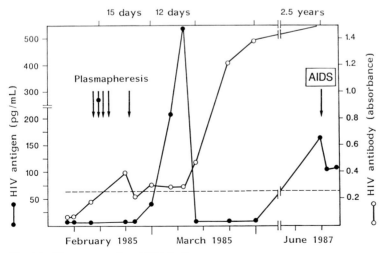

Fig. 4.1 The course of an HIV infection

complexes with them. If an excess of core-protein antibodies is produced, all the antigen will be trapped in complexes and the antigen test will become negative. At a certain point during the infection, the production of antigen is activated, resulting in an excess of antigen; thus the antigen test becomes positive again.

A prospective study of large groups of infected homosexual men has shown that the reappearance of HIV antigen in the serum of an asymptomatic individual is the precursor to the development of AIDS. A similar pattern could be seen in this patient; she was symptom-free for 2.5 years and no HIV antigen could be demonstrated. HIV antigen only reappeared when AIDS was diagnosed. With antiviral therapy (zidovudine), viral production could be reduced, as is apparent from the drop in serum level of HIV antigen following the initiation of therapy.

How can one recognize an acute or chronic HIV infection? An acute HIV infection can present symptomatically, but this is not necessarily the case. Sometimes an infection is accompanied by a flu-like syndrome. Skin abnormalities can occur and retrosternal pain combined with swallowing problems have been described as a result of *Candida* esophagitis. Encephalopathy, meningitis, and neuropathies can also occur in an acute infection. The incubation time for the flu-like syndrome varies from 1 to 4 weeks; the incubation time for the neurologic symptoms is 2–6 weeks. Because the complaints or symptoms are not specific, the case history makes an important contribution to establishing whether there is an acute HIV infection: in particular, asking about recent events which could have resulted in the transmission of the HIV (sexual contact, blood transfusion, intravenous drug abuse) can lead to the diagnosis.

As shown in Figure 4.1, the serologic diagnostics in the early phase can be helpful. HIV antigen can be demonstrated over a period of a few weeks in about 10–40% of those primarily infected. Then antibodies develop. It is not possible in all cases to demonstrate antibodies following the antigen peak, and thus a "window" phase can occur in which neither antibody nor antigen is demonstrable. IgM antibodies to HIV can only be demonstrated in about 50% of all primary infections, but no earlier than IgG antibodies, and thus they do not play a role in routine diagnosis.

It is obvious that occasionally an individual will experience an acute HIV infection without any previous serologic indications. This is why it is recommended that the antigen test and the antibody test be repeated in follow-up sera taken at intervals of several weeks in those cases in which infection is strongly suspected. If after 3 months no antibodies can be demonstrated in the third generation HIV ELISA, which can also detect HIV-2 antibodies, the patient can be regarded as not being infected. Once the HIV antibody test is positive, then it will remain positive for the rest of the patient's life.

The Structure and Replication of HIV

In order to be able to discuss the pathogenesis of HIV infections, it is essential to be aware of the structure and replication cycle of the virus.

What does the virus particle look like (Fig. 4.2)? The outside of an HIV particle is an envelope, consisting of a membrane derived from a cell, into which thumb tack–shaped objects have been inserted; these are encoded by the viral genome. This thumb tack (composed of proteins coupled to sugar groups/carbohydrate groups) consists of a head, glycoprotein 120, and a point, glycoprotein 41. This envelope contains the core proteins p17 (situated on the outside) and p24 (the innermost core protein). In the nucleus of the particle are two identical molecules of single-stranded RNA (the viral genome) and several copies of the enzyme, reverse transcriptase.

How does the virus replicate (Fig. 4.3)? The *retro*viruses, to which the HIV belongs, derive their name from the enzyme reverse transcriptase.

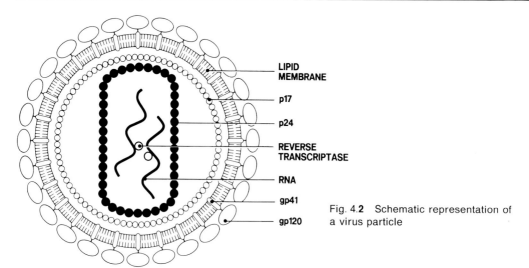

LIPID
MEMBRANE

p17

p24

REVERSE
TRANSCRIPTASE

RNA

gp41

gp120

Fig. 4.2   Schematic representation of a virus particle

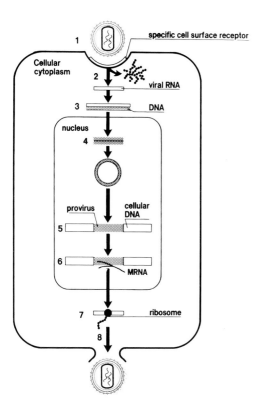

Fig. 4.3   Diagram showing replication cycle of virus

This enzyme has the unique property of being able to transcribe ribonucleic acid (RNA) into Deoxyribonucleic acid (DNA). Converting RNA into DNA is an essential step in the replication cycle of a retrovirus. Once a cell has become infected, the viral RNA is transcribed into DNA by the reverse transcriptase which was brought into the cell by the virus. The DNA is then integrated into the host cell genome; this is a "provirus." It can exist for a long time (years) before messenger RNA is produced. This is the latent phase. If the cell is "activated," the provirus will also be activated via largely unknown mechanisms, resulting in the manufacture of viral messenger RNA (mRNA), which in turn stimulates the cell to produce viral proteins. Genomic RNA is also produced. The viral proteins, together with the genomic RNA and the modified cell membrane derived from the host cell, form a new virus particle (Figs. 4.4, 4.5).

Analysis of the viral genome of HIV has revealed that, in addition to the genes that encode for structural proteins (of which the virus is composed, such as gp120, gp41, p17, and p24), other genes are also present. These code for enzymes which regulate the amount of virus produced (tat, nef, rev, protease) or the infectivity of the virus particle.

Furthermore, there are genes which code for viral proteins whose function has not yet been elucidated.

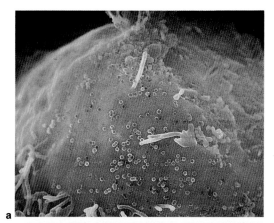

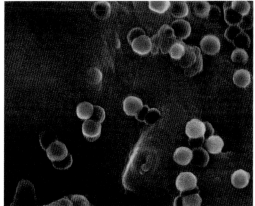

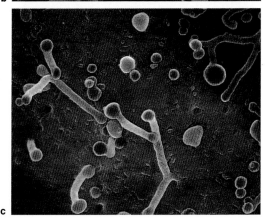

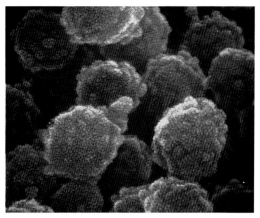

Fig. 4.**5**   A few mature HIV particles, enlarged almost 1 000 000 times. The glycoprotein projections can even be seen. This electron-microscopic technique does not allow further enlargement. The virus particles are not yet complete, but undergo a maturational process which also gives them a definitive inner structure (© Boehringer Ingelheim International GmbH; photography by L. Nilsson)

Pathogenesis

HIV uses the CD4 receptor to penetrate cells. The most important host cell is the CD4 receptor–bearing T-lymphocyte, the T-helper cell (Fig. 4.**6**). However, other CD4-positive cells, such as macrophages B cells, dendritic (antigen-presenting), and microglia cells can also become infected in vivo. The T-helper cell fulfills a central role in the regulation of the immune response. In the course of an HIV infection, functional disorders of the T-helper cell can already be established in the laboratory during the asymptomatic phase of the infection. These disorders are independent of the number of helper cells. Moreover, the number of T-helper cells gradually decreases during the infection. Ultimately, in the final stage of the illness, the existence of an immune disorder can be directly deduced from the nature of the syndrome, i.e., the occurrence of opportunistic infections.

Fig. 4.**4a–c**   The process which a cell uses to produce new viral particles involves budding; the particles free themselves *en masse* from the cell surface. Virus particles often develop on the finger-shaped protrusions. Young (red) and more mature buds (blue) are visible; in **b**, scarring can also be seen (enlargements of Fig. 4.**6**, © Boehringer Ingelheim International GmbH; photography by L. Nilsson)

The T-helper cells are probably the most important reservoir and the most important site of production of the virus. The drop in

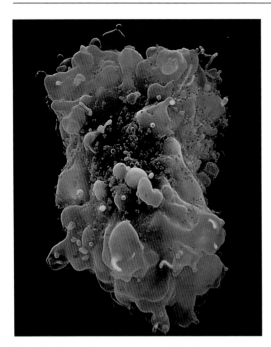

Fig. 4.**6** A major component of the immune system, a helper T-cell, can be seen to be under attack by the AIDS virus (blue). Multiple bladder- and finger-shaped protrusions of the cell can be seen (© Boehringer Ingelheim International GmbH; photography by L. Nilsson)

the number of T-helper cells is possibly due to a direct lethal effect of intracellular virus production. In vitro studies have shown that signals which are a physiological stimulus for the T-helper cell also activate the integrated provirus, with the result that the production of viral particles gets underway.

Although at a cellular level the HIV can remain latent, it would appear to be incorrect to talk in general about a latent infection, because at each phase of the HIV infection, cell-free virus can be demonstrated in serum. This illustrates that continual replication proceeds at a low level. However, in the phase of disease progression, the continual drop in the number of T-helper cells seems to be associated with a raised level of virus replication, as reflected by the increased levels of antigen and the amount of virus. This suggests that at a certain time there is a transition from a steady-state, low level of virus produc-

tion to increased virus production. Several mechanisms which operate during the infection cycle could contribute to the course described above. These mechanisms can be subdivided into viral and immunologic factors. Investigation of viruses isolated during the course of HIV infections has shown that the biological properties of the virus in a person can change in the sense that viruses acquire properties that allow them to grow in several laboratory cell lines and that cause T-helper cells to fuse. Furthermore, during the course of an infection, the virus gradually changes the composition of the membrane protein at sites aimed at by the immune response. The most important site (epitope) is situated on gp120. Early in the infection, antibodies to this gp are manufactured which retard penetration of the virus into the cells, and thus neutralize it. These neutralizing antibodies could play a role in vivo to counteract massive viral spread. By altering precisely this epitope, the virus could eventually escape the neutralizing antibodies. Even in the asymptomatic phase, functional disorders can be demonstrated at several levels of the immune apparatus (T-helper cell, B-cell response, chemotaxis of the macrophage, cytotoxic T-cell response). The extent to which certain factors are the cause or the result of the advancing immunodeficiency, and what the effects are of interaction between viral and immunologic processes, is the subject of intense investigation.

Treatment of HIV Infection

In the ideal situation, curing a person infected with HIV requires the complete abolition of all viruses from the body. This means that all proviruses should also be eliminated. In the absence of such a method, the prevention of virus production is an alternative. The first medicine to be successfully applied for this purpose on a large scale is zidovudine. The action of zidovudine, or AZT, lies in a specific interaction between the medicine and the enzyme reverse transcriptase. This enzyme incorporates the zidovudine into the growing DNA of the new provirus. Once incorporated, the zidovudine prevents further extension of the DNA molecule, so that a complete virus cannot be produced. The effect is that no further spread of the virus can occur, but the virus does remain in previously infected cells. Treatment of AIDS patients with zidovudine results in a drop in the amount of virus, an increase in the amount of T-helper cells and an extension of the life expectancy by a few years. Thus, zidovudine only yields a few extra years of life. It has been established in the laboratory that during the course of treatment with zidovudine, HIV strains develop which are insensitive to zidovudine levels attainable in vivo. It is not inconceivable that the development of resistant strains is partially to blame for the fact that zidovudine is only effective for a limited time.

Several substances have been developed whose antiviral effect is based on the same mechanism as that of zidovudine; however, their application on a large scale is prevented by serious side-effects.

In the search for new medicines, one looks to other viral enzymes such as protease. Interim results of a totally different method, in which a soluble form of CD4 was administered to patients for the purpose of surrounding released viruses with CD4 and thus preventing them from entering the cell, do not give much reason for hope.

Conclusion

It appears that the majority of all HIV-infected individuals eventually dies from an acquired immunodeficiency. The length of the period from the moment of infection to the actual development of AIDS can, however, vary considerably (from a few months to 9 years). From the above, one can deduce that the human immune system does not (yet) have a satisfactory solution to suppressing or eliminating the infection. The cytotoxic T-cell response and neutralizing antibodies, two important pillars on which the fight against other infections rests, do not appear to be capable of successfully combating an HIV infection. Two properties of the virus are partially responsible for this: the ability to remain latent in some cells and the ability to continually change those components at which the human immune response aims. Because the virus infection has direct effects on different compartments of the immune system, for many disorders it is difficult to indicate whether they are the cause or result of disease progression. An important question remains: does reactivation of virus infection occur because of the appearance of certain immunologic disorders, or do immune disorders develop because of reactivation, or are both hypotheses correct? Answers to these questions can be obtained by studying the regulation of viral replication and the role of the viral variation which occurs in relation to the immunologic parameters.

Intervention via administration of antiviral substances (zidovudine), neutralizing antibodies, and immune modulators (interferon, interleukines) can help to provide insight into the importance of the different processes in retarding or preventing progression of disease. Until a strategy has been developed which can eliminate host cells with (latent) provirus, it is impossible to actually cure the infection.

Much research in the next few years will be aimed at developing methods to eliminate HIV and at developing an effective vaccine. Until this has been achieved, the medical profession can help AIDS patients by establishing diagnosis rapidly, so that adequate treatment can be initiated early on. Furthermore, there are indications that one should examine the effect of treatment with virostatic substances of individuals in the asymptomatic stages of HIV infection, with a view to determining the extent to which progression to AIDS can be delayed or even prevented.

References

Fauci AS. The human immunodeficiency virus: infectivity and mechanisms of pathogenesis. Science 1988; 239:617–22.

Gottlieb MS, Groopman JE. Acquired immune deficiency syndrome (UCLA symposia on molecular and cellular biology). New York: Alan R Liss, 1984.

Groopman JE, Chen ISY, Essex M, Weiss RA. Human retroviruses (UCLA symposium on human retroviruses). New York: Wiley-Liss, 1989.

Ho DD, Pomerantz RJ, Kaplan JC. Pathogenesis of infection with human immunodeficiency virus. N Engl J Med 1987;317:278–86.

Levy JA. Mysteries of HIV: challenges for therapy and prevention. Nature 1988;333:519–22.

Rosenblum ML, Levy RM, Bredesen DE. AIDS and the nervous system. New York: Raven Press, 1988.

Varmus H. Retroviruses. Science 1988;240:1427–35.

5 Prevention of HIV Transmission in Diagnostic Procedures

P. J. van den Broek

Introduction

The arrival of AIDS has aroused a great deal of interest in the dangers involved in working in the health services. The hepatitis B virus (HBV) was never the source of such interest, although it does have a reputation for being the cause of occupational illness. Undoubtedly, the fact that AIDS always ends fatally is the reason so much attention has been devoted to the risks run by the health care worker. AIDS has drastically influenced work in the health services. In a way, this can be regarded as a favorable side-effect of the disease.

Particularly at the beginning, when the manner in which the disease spread was still unclear, the risks were greatly overestimated. This chapter deals first of all with a realistic estimation of the risk and discusses which materials should be considered to be infectious and how infection can occur. After a brief discussion about the basis of prevention of HIV infections in the health services, the necessary general precautions are considered. Then, in the light of these measures, imaging techniques are discussed, leading to the conclusion that alongside the general precautions, no extra measures are necessary. The final paragraph is devoted to the seropositive employee.

Danger of Infection

The human immunodeficiency virus is, as far as routes of infection are concerned, comparable to HBV. It has become clear from epidemiologic studies that the virus can be transmitted via blood, semen, cervical and vaginal secretions, and breast milk (1). Analogous to hepatitis B, all fluids present in the body normally or under pathologic conditions are considered to be infectious. The

Table 5.1 Materials which can transmit HIV

Infectious	Infectious if visibly blood-stained
Blood	Urine
Semen	Feces
Vaginal and cervical secretion	Saliva
Wound and tissue fluid	Sputum
Cerebrospinal fluid	Vomit
Amniotic fluid	Sweat
Pleural fluid	Tears
Pericardial fluid	
Peritoneal fluid	
Nasal secretion	
Synovial fluid	

virus can be demonstrated in urine, feces, tears, etc., but these excretae are not considered to be infectious unless they are visibly contaminated with blood (Table 5.1).

Transmission of HIV can occur in the health services if employees wound themselves on a sharp object such as a needle or scalpel which has been used on a patient ("pricking accident"), or if mucous membranes or broken skin are exposed to materials containing HIV. The chance of the person concerned becoming seropositive after a pricking accident which results in exposure to blood with HIV is 0.4%. This chance is maximally 0.9% (upper limit of the 95% confidence interval; 2–4). The chance of contracting hepatitis B following accidental pricking and exposure to HBV-positive blood is much greater: 6–30% (5–7). The explanation which is given for this difference is that many more virus particles are found in the blood of HBV carriers than in the majority of HIV-seropositive patients. If broken skin or mucous membranes are exposed to blood or other materials containing HIV, the chance of a seroconversion to HIV is much smaller than by accidental pricking. The actual percent chance cannot be stated precisely, because in the various prospective studies performed, no cases of infection have as yet occurred via this route. Only on the basis of information from case histories it is clear that infection via broken skin or mucous membranes is a possibility (2–4).

The size of the risk is partly determined by the prevalence of seropositive persons in the general population or patient population. In the Netherlands, there are no satisfactory data on this subject. The prevalence in an Amsterdam hospital among surgical patients who took part voluntarily in a study was 0.23% (8). The rate among pregnant women in Amsterdam who allowed themselves to be tested was 0.28% (9). The prevalence will differ strongly from place to place and according to the composition of the patient population.

Minimizing the Danger of Infection

Basically, there are two strategies for minimizing the danger of HIV infection in the health services. The first possibility is to adapt daily procedures so that the chance of infection becomes virtually nil. Using this approach to the problem, it is not necessary to take extra measures when dealing with AIDS patients or those who are known to be seropositive (10, 11). The alternative approach is only to take measures when dealing with patients who present a risk. These include patients with AIDS, AIDS-related complex, or generalized lymphadenopathy, HIV-seropositive patients and HBV carriers, as well as patients who belong to a medical or social category with a high prevalence of HIV seropositivity and HBV carriers (12). The ultimate consequence of this approach is to look for HIV antibodies in patients who have to undergo interventions carrying a certain inherent risk to the person performing them, and to take extra measures in those found to be seropositive.

Arguments presented in support of the former approach (general precautions) are: a)

the fact that it is impossible to distinguish patients at risk on the basis of appearance or on clinical grounds (13); b) the limited value of antibody determination for predicting whether someone is infectious, as there is a phase in the disease during which patients do have the virus in their blood but no antibodies (14, 15); c) the problems caused by false-positive results, burdening the patient for the rest of his or her life (16); d) the fact that general precautions also protect against other blood-borne disorders; yesterday it was hepatitits B, today it is AIDS, and tomorrow it will be something new; e) there will always be a need for general precautions, because there are many situations in which it is impossible to know whether or not the patient is seropositive.

Advocates of taking specific measures involving the testing of patients point out in particular the impracticability of general precautions because these are too time-consuming and too expensive.

In the Netherlands, the national Working group for the Prevention of Infection (WIP), in collaboration with the Health Service Advice Committee on AIDS and the National Committee to Combat AIDS (NCAB), elected to draw up guidelines with the intention of implementing general precautions* (17–20). With regard to testing patients, in the Netherlands we are bound by statements made by the government. The Health Advice Committee on AIDS and the NCAB have taken the stand that it is not permissible to test patients for the purpose of taking protective measures for health service employees (21, 22).

General Precautions

General precautions involve a broad range of activities (Table 5.2). First of all, all health

---

* The guidelines of the WIP can be obtained from the documentation center of the working group, University Hospital Leiden, Building 1, L4-P, Rijnsburgerweg 10, 2333 AA Leiden, The Netherlands, telephone: 071-226399 (from 9:00 a.m. to 1:00 p.m.).

Table 5.2   General precautions for preventing HIV transmission

Good personal hygiene
Avoidance of accidental pricking
Avoidance of contamination of broken skin and
    mucous membranes
Use of equipment for resuscitation
Sterilization and disinfection

service employees should maintain excellent personal hygiene. Everyone must wear occupational clothing, which should be changed every day. When clothing becomes stained with blood or other potentially infectious materials, the employee should immediately change into clean clothes. When there is a chance of severe contamination with infectious materials and of one's own clothing getting wet, special damp-resistant clothing should be worn. Washing and disinfecting the hands are the cornerstones of personal hygiene. Contaminated hands must always be washed with soap and water. In all other cases, disinfecting the hands with (hand) alcohol is a good alternative (23).

Sharp objects must be treated with care. The most frequent pricking accidents occur when putting a needle back into its protective sheath, when putting away unprotected needles, and when collecting garbage if needles have simply been thrown into the plastic garbage bag. The solution to this needle problem is a container made of hard plastic, with a lid, into which needles and other sharp objects can be deposited. The lid of the container allows needle and syringe to be separated. These containers should nowadays be present in large quantities in every hospital, i.e., in large numbers and in many locations so that one never has to walk too far to find one. Replacing needles in sheaths and simply throwing needles into plastic rubbish bags will thus become a thing of the past and a serious error.

When it is necessary to replace a needle in the sheath, one should either use a protective cover for the hand, or not hold the sheath in the hand (24, 25).

Infection via broken skin must be avoided by covering skin wounds well with a waterproof plaster. Gloves should be worn if one expects to be in contact with blood or other potentially infectious substances, with damaged skin or mucous membranes, with blood-stained material and instruments, and when performing procedures involving blood. When there is a possibility of being spattered or squirted with blood or infectious substances, the mucous membranes must be protected by wearing a nose-mouth mask and glasses or goggles. Ordinary glasses are also adequate, provided they completely cover the eyes.

In the hospital, equipment for artificial respiration must be ubiquitously available. For mouth to mouth resuscitation in acute situations, there should be access to equipment with a one-way valve or a stop-valve.

HIV can be inactivated by sterilization using hot air ($170\,^\circ$C), steam ($121-134\,^\circ$C), or ethylene oxide, by thermal disinfection (temperature above $80\,^\circ$C for 10 minutes), and by chemical disinfection. HIV is sensitive to many disinfectants, but in practice one must choose a substance that not only kills HIV but also HBV. This limits the possibilities to chlorine compounds (0.1% free chlorine), ethanol 70%, and glutaraldehyde 2%. Disinfection must always be preceded by cleansing, because chlorine compounds and ethanol are inactivated by organic material.

When, in spite of all precautions, there is a possibility that infection with HIV has occurred, the wound or infected skin or mucous membrane surface should be rinsed very well with water and then disinfected with 70% ethanol. If the victim has not been vaccinated against HBV, 5 mL hepatitis B immunoglobulin must be administered and vaccination initiated immediately. There is no preventive measure against HIV. In experimental animals, prophylactic administration of zidovudine over a period of time has been instigated immediately after the possible infection, but the results are disappointing. Too little experience has been gained in humans. It is advisable to take blood from the victim and to repeat this after 3, 6, and possibly 12 months. HIV antibodies are only determined in the last sample drawn. If this investigation proves positive, then the previous samples are also analyzed, particularly the first one, to determine whether one is dealing with an occupational disease (26).

Risks in Imaging Diagnostic Procedures

Following the above outline of general precautions, one should look at whether unusual situations arise in imaging diagnostics, for which these general measures are inadequate. The greatest risk lies in the angiographic technique. The radiologist should be dressed in surgical garments including a nose-mouth mask. Considering that there is a chance of blood being spattered, it is strongly advised that glasses be worn. Further measures seem to be superfluous. The person assisting with the procedure should take similar precautions.

Another job accompanied by high risk is the examination of trauma patients. Contact with blood is usually unavoidable. Only general precautions can offer a solution here, because rarely is anything about the patient known.

Imaging diagnostics often involve giving injections. Provided the needles are disposed of in the correct way, there is no exceptional risk. The same is true for needles used for diagnostic punctures, e.g., under the guidance of ultrasonography. After use, the ultrasonography head must be cleaned and disinfected with 70% ethanol.

The Seropositive Employee

Until now, only the danger that patients present to health service employees has been considered, but what is the risk the other way around? There are a number of examples of hepatitis B epidemics in which the doctor was the source of infection (27–29). It is, therefore, not inconceivable that a patient might be infected by a health care professional. This danger is particularly real when he or she can wound him- or herself when assisting a patient, e.g., with a needle-prick or by cutting him- or herself on the patient's teeth. In general, being a carrier of HBV is not considered reason enough to forbid someone from performing his or her duties. But such a person must take extra precautions, such as wearing double gloves when carrying out procedures. This same policy could be implemented for HIV-seropositive employees.

References

1. CDC. Update: universal precautions for prevention of transmission of HIV, Hepatitis B virus and other blood-borne pathogens in health-care settings. JAMA 1988; 260:462–5.
2. Houweling H, Coutinho RA. Is AIDS een beroepsrisico voor de (para)medische beroepsgroepen? Ned Tijdschr Geneeskd 1987; 131: 2183–6.
3. CDC. AIDS–HIV update: AIDS and HIV infection among health care workers. JAMA 1988; 259: 2817–21.
4. Marcus R et al. Surveillance of health care workers exposed to blood from patients infected with the HIV. N Engl J Med 1988; 319: 1118–23.
5. Grady et al. Hepatitis B immune globulin for accidental exposures among medical personnel: final report of a multicenter controlled trial. J Infect Dis 1978; 138:625–38.
6. Seeff LB. Type B hepatitis after needle-stick exposure: prevention with hepatitis B immune globulin. Ann Intern Med 1978; 88:285–93.
7. Werner BG, Grady GF. Accidental hepatitis-B-surface-antigen-positive inoculations. Ann Intern Med 1982; 97:367–9.
8. Leentvaar-Kuipers A et al. HIV-beroepsrisico van snijdende specialisten en operatierkamermedewerkers in het Sint Lucas Ziekenhuis te Amsterdam. Ned Tijdschr Geneeskd 1989; 133:2388–91.
9. Coutinho RA et al. HIV-prevalentie bij zwangeren in drie poliklinieken in Amsterdam. Ned Tijdschr Geneeskd 1989; 133:978–80.
10. CDC. Recommendations for prevention of HIV transmission in health-care settings. MMWR 1987; 36:suppl 2S.
11. CDC. Update: universal precautions for prevention of transmission of human immunodeficiency virus, Hepatitis B virus, and other bloodborne pathogens in health-care settings. MMWR 1988; 37:377–87.

12. Speller et al. Acquired immune deficiency syndrome: recommendations of a working party of the Hospital Infection Society. J Hosp Infect 1990;15:7–34.
13. Kelen GD et al. Unrecognized human immunodeficiency virus infection in emergency department patients. N Engl J Med 1988;318:1645–50.
14. Imagawa DT et al. Human immunodeficiency virus type 1 infection in homosexual men who remain seronegative for prolonged periods. N Engl J Med 1989;320:1458–62.
15. Horsburgh CR et al. Duration of human immunodeficiency virus infection before detection of antibody. Lancet 1989;2:637–40.
16. Verbrugh HA. Screening van patiënten op HIV-infectie ter preventie van besmetting van zorgverleners in ziekenhuizen. Ned Tijdschr Geneeskd 1987;131:2207–8.
17. WIP. Richtlijn ter voorkoming van HIV-besmetting in de intramurale gezondheidszorg. Richtlijn 34, Leiden, 1988.
18. WIP. HIV-infectiepreventie in laboratoria. Richtlijn 42, Leiden, 1989.
19. WIP. HIV-infektiepreventie in de chirurgie. Richtlijn 43, Leiden, 1990.
20. WIP. HIV-infektiepreventie in de pathologische anatomie. Richtlijn 44, Leiden, 1990.
21. Gezondheidsraad. AIDS-problematiek in Nederland. Richtlijnen voor groepsonderzoek en adviezen voor preventie. Den Haag, 1986.
22. Gezondheidsraad. Maatregelen om ziekenhuispersoneel tijdens de beroepsuitoefening te beschermen tegen besmetting met de verwekker van AIDS. Den Haag, 1988.
23. Mouton RP. Consensus preventie ziekenhuisinfekties. Ned Tijdschr Geneeskd 1990;134:231–5.
24. Nixon AD et al. Simple device to prevent accidental needle-prick injuries. Lancet 1986;1:888–9.
25. Broek van den PJ. Preventie van prikongevallen. Ned Tijdschr Geneeskd 1987;131:2187–8.
26. WIP. Besmetting met bloed: preventie van prikongevallen en handelwijze na besmetting met bloed. Richtlijn 36, Leiden, 1989.
27. Grob PJ et al. Cluster of hepatitis B transmitted by a physician. Lancet 1981;2:1218–20.
28. Carl M et al. Interruption of hepatitis B transmission by modification of a gynaecologist's surgical technique. Lancet 1982;1:731–3.
29. Welch J et al. Hepatitis B infections after gynaecological surgery. Lancet 1989;1:205–6.

6 Clinical Neurology of AIDS

P. Portegies

Introduction

In patients with HIV-1 infection, the nervous system is commonly affected (1–3). Neurologic involvement occurs in at least 40% of patients, who usually already meet the CDC's clinical criteria for AIDS, and it is the presenting manifestation in 10% of HIV-1–infected patients. At autopsy, 80–90% are found to have neuropathologic abnormalities.

The spectrum of neurologic complications includes opportunistic infections, neoplasms, and complications related to or caused by the HIV-1 itself. The most common neurologic manifestations will be discussed here; their treatments are summarized in Table 6.1.

Opportunistic Infections

Cerebral Toxoplasmosis

Cerebral toxoplasmosis is the leading cause of focal brain disease in AIDS patients, and has a prevalence of 3–40%, depending on the seroprevalence. Cerebral toxoplasmosis is the presenting opportunistic infection in at least 5% of the AIDS patient population (4).

Clinically patients with cerebral toxoplasmosis present with constitutional symptoms, headache and fever, followed by focal neurologic abnormalities, including focal seizures, aphasia, hemiparesis, and homonymous hemianopia, depending on the localization of the lesions (5). This combination of focal

Table 6.**1** Treatment scheme of neurological manifestations

Neurological manifestations	Treatment
Opportunistic infections	
Cerebral toxoplasmosis	sulfadiazine and pyrimethamine (clindamycin)
Cryptococcal meningitis	amphotericin B and flucytosine (fluconazole, itraconazole)
PML	cytarabine?
CMV infections	ganciclovir (DHPG)
Tumors	
Primary CNS lymphoma	radiation therapy (surgery?, chemotherapy?)
Lymphomatous meningitis	intrathecal methotrexate
CNS Kaposi's sarcoma	?
HIV-1 – related manifestations	
AIDS dementia complex	zidovudine
Vacuolar myelopathy	none
Aseptic meningitis	none
Peripheral neuropathics	
DSPN	symptomatic: carbamazepine, amitriptyline, phenytoin
AIDP, CIDP	plasmapheresis, corticosteroids
MM	none
Myopathies	
Polymyositis	corticosteroids?
Zidovudine-myopathy	temporary interruption of zidovudine treatment

abnormalities and signs of a global enceph-alopathy is very suggestive.

Brain imaging is very important in es-tablishing the diagnosis. CT scan normally reveals multiple hypodense areas, usually with mass effect, and contrast enhancement (ring pattern or irregular nodular). MRI is more sensitive in detecting lesions.

In AIDS patients with suspected cerebral toxoplasmosis, based on clinical findings and CT-scan abnormalities, empirical treatment is justifiable, reserving brain biopsy for atyp-ical or refractory cases. The most effective therapy is a combination of pyrimethamine (50 mg daily) and sulfadiazine (6–8 g daily) (6). Oral folinic acid is given to prevent hematologic side effects. Six weeks induction treatment has to be followed by lifelong maintenance therapy (same combination or monotherapy with pyrimethamine). Clinda-mycin may represent an alternative therapy for sulfadiazine. Corticosteroids may be used for lesions associated with edema and mass effect.

Cryptococcal Meningitis

Cryptococcal meningitis is the most common mycotic infection involving the nervous sys-tem in patients with HIV infection. The prevalence of this life-threatening opportu-nistic infection among AIDS patients is 2–7.5%.

Clinically the disease manifests as sub-acute or chronic meningitis with headache, altered mentation, and fever. Headache may become severe, with nausea and vomiting. Neck stiffness is frequently absent. Papille-dema and 6th-nerve palsy may be present (7).

The diagnosis is based on cerebrospinal fluid (CSF) analysis: mild mononuclear pleocytosis and an elevated protein level may be present, and the fungus can be detected in india-ink preparation. Cryptococcal antigen is nearly always positive in the CSF and serum, as are fungal cultures of CSF.

Standard therapy with amphotericin B given intravenously (0.3 mg/kg/day) with or without oral flucytosine (150 mg/kg/day) is effective in about 60% of cases (8). Relapses are frequent, so maintenance treatment (after 6–8 weeks of induction) with amphotericin B (0.7–1.5 mg/kg each week) is recommended. Itraconazole and fluconazole, new antifungal oral triazole drugs, appear to be attractive alternatives to amphotericin (9).

Cytomegalovirus Encephalitis/Polyradiculitis

CMV encephalitis. This disease has no typical clinical presentation. Progressive dementia (indistinguishable from AIDS dementia com-plex) or focal abnormalities may be present, but many patients are asymptomatic. Some-times the virus can be isolated from the CSF, but often the identification of CMV is based on typical intranuclear inclusions of identi-fication of CMV antigens by immuno-cytochemistry, or both, at neuropathologic examination (10). The relative importance of CMV infection in many cases is unclear and CMV often coexists with other infectious agents.

CT scan may reveal subependymal en-hancement compatible with ventriculitis. There is no effective treatment for CMV encephalitis.

CMV polyradiculitis (or CMV polyradiculo-(myelo)pathy). This disease is an uncommon complication in patients with AIDS. Cytomegalovirus has been mentioned as the causative agent. Patients present with a pro-gressive, flaccid paraparesis, with sphincter disturbances, irradiating leg pain, or both. Reflexes in the legs are low or absent; usually sensory disturbances are mild (11). CSF analysis shows a pleocytosis (with predom-inance of polymorphonuclear leukocytes), an elevated protein level, and a positive culture for CMV. Sometimes myelographic exami-nation shows thickened, adherent lumbar nerve roots (12). Treatment with ganciclovir, also called DHPG, started early in the course of the disease, may stop progression or even cause some improvement (13).

Progressive Multifocal Leukoencephalopathy

PML is a subacute demyelinating disease resulting from infection of oligodendrocytes by a papovavirus called the JC virus. The JC virus is almost ubiquitous in adults all over the world. Seroconversion occurs in childhood, usually without producing disease. PML occurs almost exclusively in immunocompromised patients, and is estimated to occur in up to 4% of patients with AIDS.

The onset of the disease is usually insidious; the symptoms and signs suggest multifocal disease. Hemiparesis, visual field defects, cortical blindness, aphasia, ataxia, and dementia may occur. Headaches and seizures are rare, and there are no signs of raised intracranial pressure. The disease evolves relentlessly until the patient dies, usually within 4 to 6 months (14). However, stabilization or spontaneous remissions have been described.

The CSF is generally normal. CT scan of the brain shows hypodense nonenhancing white matter lesions. With MRI high signal intensity, lesions are found in the white matter (15).

Treatment of PML has been unsuccessful, despite occasional reports of a positive response to cytarabine.

Tumors

Primary lymphomas of the central nervous system. These tumors are uncommon (approximately 5% of patients with AIDS) but are second to cerebral toxoplasmosis as a cause of intracranial mass lesion. Patients with primary CNS lymphoma present with headache, seizures, altered mental status, and focal neurologic deficits (16). CT scan reveals hypodense lesions with irregular, nodular, or ringlike enhancement after administration of contrast (in 50% of cases, lesions are multiple). Despite some improvement with radiation therapy, the prognosis for AIDS patients with primary CNS lymphoma is dismal.

Lymphomatous meningitis (or leptomeningeal lymphoma). This affliction causes headache, encephalopathy, cranial nerve palsies, and spinal root dysfunction. Cytological examination of the CSF is the single most useful test for leptomeningeal lymphoma and intrathecal chemotherapy with methotrexate is the primary treatment (17).

Only a few cases of **Kaposi's sarcoma** metastatic to the brain have been published.

Neurological Syndromes Caused by or Related to HIV-1

AIDS Dementia Complex

One of the most common neurological syndromes in patients with AIDS is the AIDS dementia complex (ADC) of HIV-1 encephalopathy, which is directly related to infection of the brain with the HIV-1 (18). Without treatment, at least a third of all patients with AIDS eventually develop a mild or severe form of ADC. Clinically ADC is characterized by abnormalities in cognition, motor performance, and behavior. Usually the onset of the syndrome is insidious. With time, progression to moderate or severe global dementia occurs in all patients (19).

Neuropsychological testing reveals abnormalities conforming to a "subcortical dementia," with slowing of both mental and motor functions. CT and MRI show widened cortical sulci and enlarged ventricles. MRI shows white matter abnormalities. Several CSF abnormalities have been reported in patients with ADC, but HIV-1-p24 antigen detection and increased beta-2-microglobulin levels correlate best with clinical neurologic status (20). The pathologic abnormalities are most prominent in the central white matter and deep, gray structures (basal ganglia, thalamus, and brain stem) and include diffuse pallor of the white matter and multinucleate cell encephalitis with perivascular and parenchymal infiltrates. Some beneficial effects of zidovudine treatment in patients with ADC have been described, and since the introduction of zidovudine the incidence of ADC has declined (21, 22).

Vacuolar Myelopathy

Vacuolar myelopathy has been reported in 20–25% of AIDS cases. Clinically the syndrome is characterized by a spastic paraparesis and sensory ataxia, sometimes with urinary incontinence, and is associated with AIDS dementia complex in 60% of cases. Pathologic changes in the spinal cord are most prominent in the thoracic cord and closely mimic the pathology of subacute combined degeneration of the spinal cord (23). Although HIV has been cultured from the spinal cord, the etiologic agent and the pathogenetic mechanisms of this vacuolar myelopathy remain uncertain. Other infectious causes (CMV, HSV) and lymphomatous meningitis have to be excluded.

Aseptic Meningitis

An acute illness with headache, fever, and meningeal signs has been described at the time of seroconversion and in later stages (CDC IV-A) of HIV-1 infection. Cranial nerve involvement (usually of the 7th) and long-tract involvement have been noted. Most cases have a self-limited monophasic course, but the syndrome tends to recur. All patients, by definition, have a CSF pleocytosis, and HIV can be cultured from the CSF in the majority of these cases (24).

Peripheral Neuropathies

Besides herpes zoster infection affecting spinal or cranial nerves and CMV polyradiculitis, three major types of peripheral neuropathies of uncertain etiology have been described in patients with HIV-1 infection: 1) distal symmetric peripheral neuropathy, 2) acute and chronic inflammatory demyelinating polyradiculoneuropathy, and 3) mononeuropathy multiplex (25, 26).

Distal symmetric peripheral neuropathy (DSPN). This is the most common type, occurring in 10–25% of patients (CDC class IV-A, or AIDS). The most frequent symptoms are paresthesias, pain, and dysesthesias affecting the feet. Ankle reflexes are absent;

weakness is mild and affects only the intrinsic foot muscles. Although HIV has been isolated from peripheral nerves, the etiology remains unclear. Treatment is limited to providing symptomatic relief with tricyclic antidepressants and anticonvulsants. The effect of zidovudine has not yet been defined.

Acute inflammatory demyelinating polyradiculoneuropathy (AIDP—clinically indistinguishable from the Guillain–Barré syndrome) and **chronic inflammatory demyelinating polyradiculoneuropathy** (CIDP). These usually occur in the early stages of HIV-1 infection. Clinical manifestations include weakness, areflexia, and minor sensory symptoms. CSF abnormalities include a pleocytosis and an elevated protein level. Usually the clinical course is favorable. Most of these patients recover spontaneously or show improvement after plasmapheresis or treatment with corticosteroids.

Mononeuropathy multiplex (MM). Characterized by sensory and motor deficits in the distributions of multiple spinal, cranial, or peripheral nerves, MM is associated with CDC class IV-A and AIDS. CSF analysis reveals both pleocytosis and elevated protein level. Electrophysiologic and pathologic studies suggest axonal neuropathy. The majority of patients with MM recover spontaneously.

Myopathies

Polymyositis. This myopathy has been described in all stages of HIV-1 infection. Patients presented with myalgias, proximal weakness, and elevated serum creatine phosphokinase. Muscle biopsies showed fiber necrosis and variable inflammatory infiltrates. Some patients showed marked improvement with corticosteroids (27). *Pyomyositis* has also been described in AIDS.

Zidovudine-associated myopathy. This occurs in a minority of patients who have been treated with zidovudine for at least 9–12 months. Muscle tenderness and weakness are preceded by creatine phosphokinase elevation. Pathologically "ragged, red" fibers, indicative of abnormal mitochondria, coexist with inflammatory changes (28). Temporary interruption of zidovudine, prednisone, or nonsteroidal anti-inflammatory drugs may lead to improvement. However there is still controversy about the causal link (29).

References

1. Snider WD, Simpson DM, Nielsen S, et al. Neurological complications of acquired immune deficiency syndrome: analysis of 50 patients. Ann Neurol 1983; 14:403–18.
2. McArthur JC. Neurologic manifestations of AIDS. Medicine 1987; 66:407–37.
3. De Gans J, Portegies P. Neurological complications of infection with human immunodeficiency virus type 1: a review of literature and 241 cases. Clin Neurol Neurosurg 1989; 91:199–219.
4. Luft BJ, Remington JS. Toxoplasmosis of the central nervous system. In: Remington JS, Schwartz MN, eds. Current clinical topics in infectious diseases, vol 6. New York: McGraw-Hill, 1985:315–58.
5. Navia BA, Petito CK, Gold JWM, Cho ES, Jordan BD, Price RW. Cerebral toxoplasmosis complicating the acquired immune deficiency syndrome: clinical and neuropathological findings in 27 patients. Ann Neurol 1986; 224–38.
6. Leport C, Raffi F, Matheron S, et al. Treatment of central nervous system toxoplasmosis with pyrimethamine/sulfadiazine combination in 35 patients with the acquired immunodeficiency syndrome. Am J Med 1988; 84:94–100.
7. Dismukes WE. Cryptococcal meningitis in patients with AIDS. J Infect Dis 1988; 157:624–8.
8. Dismukes WE, Cloud G, Gallis H, et al. Treatment of cryptococcal meningitis with combination amphotericin B and flucytosine for four as compared with six weeks. N Engl J Med 1987; 317:334–41.
9. Gans J de, Eeftinck Schattenkerk JKM, Ketel RJ van. Itraconazole as maintenance treatment for cryptococcal meningitis in the acquired immune deficiency syndrome. Br Med J 1988; 296:339.
10. Morgello S, Cho ES, Nielsen S, Devinsky O, Petito CK. Cytomegalovirus encephalitis in patients with acquired immunodeficiency syndrome: an autopsy study of 30 cases and a review of the literature. Hum Pathol 1987; 18:289–97.
11. Eidelberg D, Sotrel A, Vogel H, Walker P, Kleefield J, Crumpacker CS. Progressive polyradiculopathy in acquired immune deficiency syndrome. Neurology 1986; 36:912–6.
12. Borgstein BJ, Koster PA, Portegies P, Peeters FLM. Myelography in patients with acquired immunodeficiency syndrome. Neuroradiology 1989; 31:326–30.
13. Gans J de, Portegies P, Tiessens G, Troost D, Danner SA, Lange MJA. Therapy for cytomegalovirus polyradiculomyelitis in patients with AIDS: treatment with ganciclovir. AIDS 1990; 4:421–5.
14. Berger JR, Kaszovitz B, Post MJD, Dickinson G. Progressive multifocal leukoencephalopathy associated with human immunodeficiency virus infection. Ann Intern Med 1987; 107:78–87.
15. Mark AS, Atlas SW. Progressive multifocal leukoencephalopathy in patients with AIDS: appearance on MR images. Radiology 1989; 173:517–20.
16. So YT, Beckstead JH, Davis RL. Primary central nervous system lymphoma in acquired immune deficiency syndrome: a clinical and pathological study. Ann Neurol 1986; 20:566–72.
17. So YT, Choucair A, Davis RL, et al. Neoplasms of the central nervous system in acquired immunodeficiency syndrome. In: Rosenblum ML, Levy RM, Bredesen DE, eds. AIDS and the nervous system. New York: Raven Press, 1988:285–300.
18. Price RW, Brew B, Sidtis J, et al. The brain in AIDS: central nervous system HIV-1 infection and the AIDS dementia complex. Science 1988; 239:586–92.
19. Navia BA, Jordan BD, Price RW. The AIDS dementia complex: I. clinical features. Ann Neurol 1986; 19:517–24.
20. Portegies P, Epstein LG, Hung STA, Gans J de, Goudsmit J. Human immunodeficiency virus type 1 antigen in cerebrospinal fluid: correlation with clinical neurologic status. Arch Neurol 1989; 46:261–4.
21. Schmitt FA, Bigley JW, McKinnis R, et al. Neuropsychological outcome of zidovudine (AZT) treatment of patients with AIDS and AIDS-related complex. N Engl J Med 1988; 319:1573–8.
22. Portegies P, Gans J de, Lange JMA, Derix MMA, Speelman JD, Bakker M, Danner SA, Goudsmit J. Declining incidence of AIDS dementia complex after introduction of zidovudine treatment. Br Med J 1989; 299:819–21.
23. Petito CK, Navia BA, Cho ES, Jordan BD, George DC, Price RW. Vacuolar myelopathy pathologically resembling subacute degeneration in patients with the acquired immunodeficiency syndrome. N Engl J Med 1985; 312:874–9.
24. Ho DD, Sarngadharan MG, Resnick L, et al. Primary human T-lymphotropic virus type III infection. Ann Intern Med 1985; 103:880–3.

25. De la Monte SM, Gabuzda DH, Ho DD, et al. Peripheral neuropathy in the acquired immunodeficiency syndrome. Ann Neurol 1988;23:485–92.

26. Dalakas MC, Pezeshkpour GH. Neuromuscular diseases associated with human immunodeficiency virus infection. Ann Neurol 1988;23 (suppl):S38–S48.

27. Dalakas MC, Pezeshkpour GH, Gravell M, Sever JL. Polymyositis associated with AIDS retrovirus. JAMA 1986;256:2381–3.

28. Dalakas MC, Illa I, Pezeshkpour GH, Laukaitis JP, Cohen B, Griffin JL. Mitochondrial myopathy caused by long-term zidovudine therapy. N Engl J Med 1990;322:1098–105.

29. Simpson DM. Myopathy associated with human immunodeficiency virus (HIV) but not with zidovudine. Ann Intern Med 1988;109:842.

7 CT in Intracranial Manifestations of AIDS

P. A. Koster

CT findings in AIDS patients with neurologic complications can be divided into the following groups:

1. atrophy
2. mass lesions
3. white matter lesions
4. leptomeningeal and/or ependymal disease

Atrophy

Cerebral atrophy is a very general finding and is present in about 40% of AIDS patients with neurologic symptoms (2). The etiology of atrophy has not yet been completely elucidated, but it is assumed that there is a direct relationship with the neurotropic human immunodeficiency virus (HIV), considered to be responsible for so-called subacute or HIV encephalitis. When found in combination with the clinical picture of dementia, this disorder is considered to be part of the AIDS dementia complex (ADC). At a later stage, white matter abnormalities also develop.

Atrophy is often seen in patients with HIV encephalitis following cerebral toxoplasmosis and also in cases of encephalitis caused by the cytomegalovirus (CMV), herpes simplex virus (HSV), and (very rarely) varicella-zoster virus (VZV; 2, 3, 4, 5, 6).

The enlargement of fluid spaces, both central and peripheral, can be seen in CT (Fig. 7.1).

Severe atrophy is, however, not necessarily indicative of dementia.

Mass Lesions

Intracranial mass lesions are a common finding in AIDS patients. The most frequently occurring abnormalities are toxoplasmosis and the primary intracerebral lymphoma. Other abnormalities such as intracranial Kaposi's sarcoma, *Candida* abscess, bacterial abscess, tuberculoma, and cryptococcoma are extremely rare.

Toxoplasmosis

Toxoplasmosis is found in about 20% of AIDS patients with neurologic complications (7). It thus forms the most frequently occurring intracranial lesion, and moreover, it can be treated quite successfully. It is, therefore, important that the diagnosis be established at an early stage. CT generally shows several focal lesions in the cerebrum. The lesions are usually hypodense and surrounded by a large amount of edema, giving rise to mass effects. Administration of intravenous contrast is almost always followed by enhancement, either ring-shaped (Fig. 7.2), or in the form of irregular nodules (8, 9).

Sometimes (5%) no enhancement is observed following contrast administration (8). It is assumed that the lack of enhancement is related to the disturbed immune system of the patient, resulting in little or no capsule formation around the toxoplasmosis abscess. This would be indicative of a poor prognosis (11).

Sometimes enhancement of the ventricular ependyma and/or the leptomeninges can be observed (10; Fig. 7.3).

The localization of the toxoplasmosis foci is not characteristic, although some authors do refer to the area of the basal nuclei as a preferential site (1, 11; Fig. 7.4).

If one is dealing with a solitary focus, this may indeed be due to toxoplasmosis; however, one should be aware of the possibility of lymphoma.

Considering the high incidence of toxoplasmosis in AIDS patients, it would seem

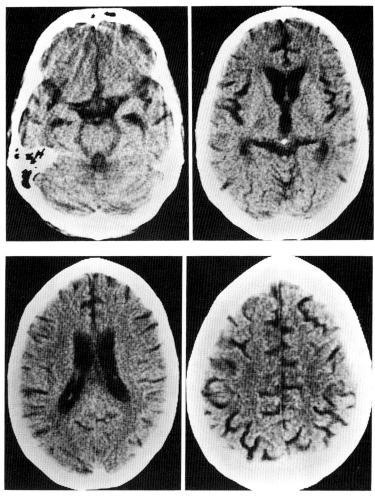

Fig. 7.1   Atrophy in a 30-year-old man. Enlargement of the ventricle system and peripheral fluid spaces

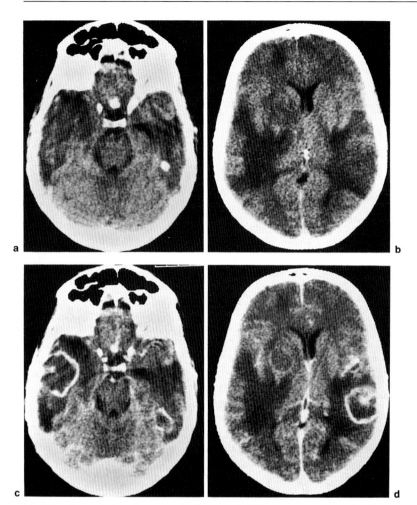

Fig. 7.2   Several toxoplasmosis lesions. **a**, **b** Without contrast; **c**, **d** with contrast: a pair of ring-shaped enhanced lesions with considerable edema

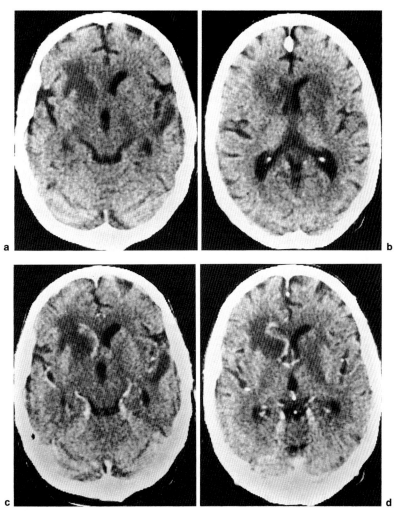

Fig. 7.3 Atypical toxoplasmosis localized subependymally. **a, b** Without contrast; **c, d** with contrast: periventricular enhancement around left anterior horn

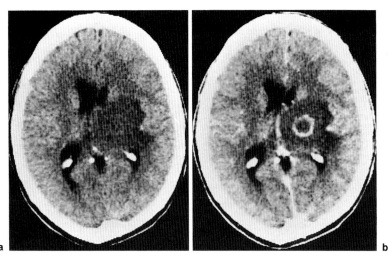

a   b

Fig. 7.**4**   Solitary toxoplasmosis lesion in the region of the basal ganglia. **a** Without contrast; **b** with contrast: target lesion surrounded by edema

justified to initiate a trial treatment with antitoxoplasmosis therapy when CT reveals one or more focal lesions (12, 13). If toxoplasmosis is involved, the abnormalities will show a definite improvement within 2 weeks of therapy, but may take 3 to 6 months to disappear completely (1, 12). Calcifications often remain, as well as signs of atrophy and small gliotic scars (2; Fig. 7.**8**).

Primary Intracerebral Lymphoma

Primary intracerebral lymphoma is the second most important category of cerebral mass lesions in AIDS patients; its incidence is considerably lower than that of toxoplasmosis; in large series, incidences of 1–2% have been found in patients with neurologic symptoms (2, 7).

There are definite differences between primary intracerebral lymphoma in AIDS and in non-AIDS patients. In AIDS patients, multiple lesion are seen in about 50% whereas this is hardly ever the case in non-AIDS patients (14, 15). The CT image is also different: in AIDS patients the lymphoma generally manifests as a hypodense mass, with more or less ring-shaped enhancement (Figs. 7.**5**, 7.**6**), while in non-AIDS patients, it

is usually an isodense or hyperdense mass, which enhances homogeneously and intensely following the administration of contrast. In AIDS patients, the lesions are often localized peripherally; in non-AIDS patients often periventricularly (5, 9, 14).

Several cases have been described in which the CT scan did not show focal abnormalities, while autopsy revealed the presence of lymphoma localizations (1, 7, 14).

A possible explanation is that CT findings in primary intracerebral lymphoma are not specific and cannot always be differentiated from toxoplasmosis.

Other Mass Lesions

While fungal infections occur frequently in patients with AIDS, it is very rare to find an intracranial abscess resulting from a fungus (*Candida albicans* or *Cryptococcus*).

Abscesses as a result of tuberculosis have indeed been described in the literature but are very rare.

CT in such abnormalities is not specific; generally, a hypodense lesion is seen which enhances roughly in the form of a ring and which is surrounded by a certain amount of edema (2, 8, 16).

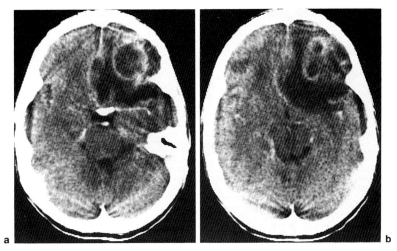

Fig. 7.**5** Primary intracerebral lymphoma. With contrast: slightly enhanced lesion with edema in the right frontal region

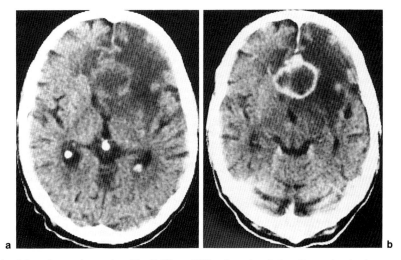

Fig. 7.**6** Primary intracerebral lymphoma (see also Fig. 7.**10**). **a** Without contrast; **b** with contrast: ring-shaped enhanced lesion in the median line with central necrosis and surrounding edema

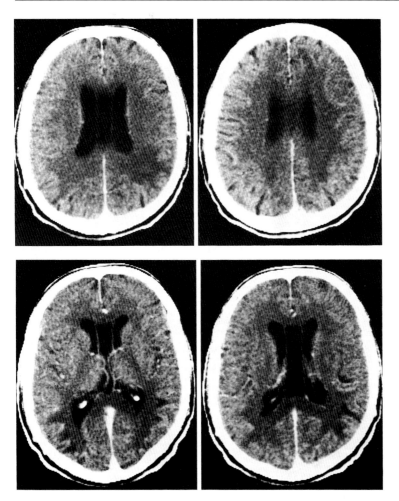

Fig. 7.**7**   HIV encephalitis in a 43-year-old man with AIDS dementia complex. Symmetrically localized white matter abnormalities, bilaterally in the parieto-occipital region and in the centrum semiovale. N.B. Cavum septi pellucidi

Intracranial metastases of Kaposi's sarcoma are extremely scarce, just like the above-mentioned abnormalities. CT demonstrates lesions which enhance after the administration of contrast and which otherwise have no specific features.

White Matter Lesions

Human Immunodeficiency Virus (HIV) Encephalitis

The most frequent cause of white matter abnormalities is HIV encephalitis. CT demonstrates hypodensity in the periventricular white matter and in the centrum semiovale, with a fairly symmetrical distribution (Figs. 7.**7**, 7.**8**). The abnormalities are confined to the white matter, and there is no question of mass effect or enhancement following the administration of contrast.

Furthermore, CT only reveals abnormalities at a late stage and is significantly less sensitive than MRI in diagnosing white matter lesions (3, 17).

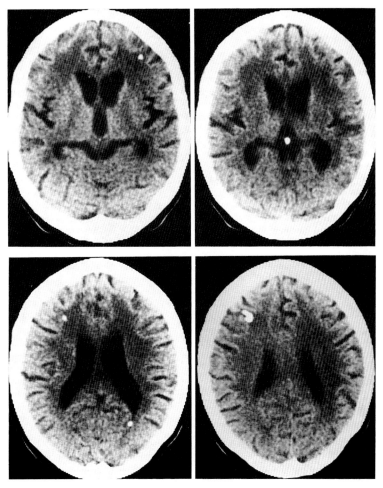

Fig. 7.**8**   HIV encephalitis in a 29-year-old man with AIDS dementia complex. Extensive white matter abnormalities; also atrophy and calcifications due to previous toxoplasmosis

Histologically, the white matter lesions in HIV encephalitis are based on areas of demyelinization, focal inflammation with infiltration of macrophages and vacuolization. The typical feature consists of multinucleate giant cells (4, 18). As already discussed, the HIV virus is responsible for the AIDS dementia complex. By applying zidovudine (AZT) therapy, the incidence of ADC has been reduced (19) and there is also a possibility of a reduction in white matter abnormalities (17).

Progressive Multifocal Leukoencephalopathy (PML)

A second important cause of white matter lesions is the JC papovavirus, the pathogen involved in progressive multifocal leukoencephalopathy. PML is clinically characterized by a rapidly progressive dementia syndrome which differs from ADC. The average survival time after establishing a diagnosis is about 3 months. PML is a relatively rare finding with an incidence of 2–4% (7, 20).

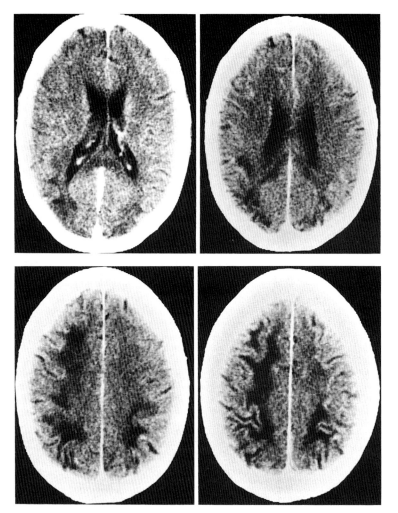

Fig. 7.**9** Progressive multifocal leukoencephalopathy in a 48 year-old man. Asymmetric white matter abnormalities spreading into the gray matter

CT demonstrates decreased density of the white matter located usually in the parieto-occipital area, where there are sometimes minor signs of mass effect. Eventually, the gray matter also becomes affected by abnormality. Following the administration of contrast, there is no visible enhancement. The lesions (Fig. 7.**9**) are generally localized in focal zones, in contrast to white matter lesions in HIV encephalitis (17) Histologically, the abnormalities in PML are due to damage to the oligodendrocytes caused by the JC virus, resulting in demyelinization, minimal edema, and ultimately necrosis.

Cytomegalovirus (CMV) Encephalitis

Although a fairly large percentage of AIDS patients is infected with cytomegalovirus, neurologic manifestations related to CMV are relatively rare. The CMV encephalitis can proceed asymptomatically and can seldom be demonstrated using CT (22).

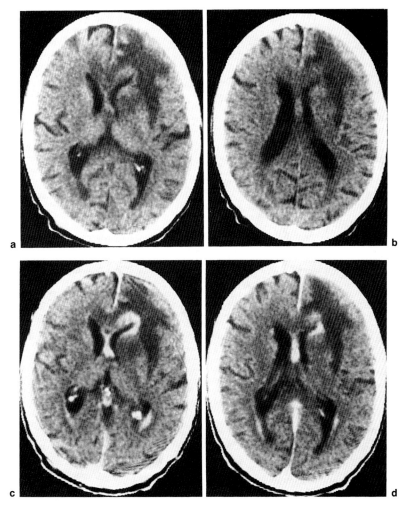

Fig. 7.**10**   Malignant lymphoma localized subependymally (see also Fig. 7.**6**). **a, b** Without contrast; **c, d** with contrast: enhancement along the ventricular ependyma spreading into the corpus callosum

Leptomeningeal and Ependymal Disease

Aseptic Meningitis

Aseptic meningitis is caused by the HIV virus and presents in 7% of AIDS patients with neurologic symptomatology (7). CT does not reveal any abnormalities in these patients, with the exception of aspecific findings such as atrophy and/or white matter lesions. The diagnosis is established on the basis of CSF analysis and the clinical status.

Cryptococcal Meningitis

Cryptococcal meningitis is a life-threatening complication in AIDS patients, occurring in about 10% of cases (7). Again, in this form of meningitis, no leptomeningeal enhancement can be seen in CT, as described in non-AIDS patients with meningitis.

Recently, CT abnormalities have been described in patients with cryptococcal meningitis; in the region of the basal nuclei, small, hypodense, nonenhancing lesions were seen, following the course of the perforating arteries (Virchow–Robin spaces). Histologic analysis revealed that these abnormalities consisted of small cysts with cryptococci and little or no inflammatory reaction (21).

Other Infections

Tuberculous meningitis is extremely rare and no specific abnormalities can be seen in CT.

A CMV infection can produce an image of ventriculitis/ependymitis, which appears in CT as a periventricular enhancement following administration of contrast (22). Ependymal lesions can also be seen in toxoplasmosis (Fig. 7.3).

Finally, one should mention the leptomeningeal and/or ependymal spread of the malignant lymphoma; here, CT sometimes reveals enhancement of the leptomeninges or of the ventricular ependyma (Fig. 7.10).

Conclusion

In the management of AIDS patients with neurologic symptoms, CT plays an important part in detecting intracranial mass lesions, most of which are caused by toxoplasmosis.

CT is of limited value in the demonstration of white matter lesions (MRI is a more sensitive modality), leptomeningeal and ependymal disease, and cerebral atrophy.

References

1. Levy RM, Bredesen DE, Rosenblum ML. Neurological manifestations of the acquired immunodeficiency syndrome (AIDS): experience at UCSF and review of the literature. J Neurosurg 1985;62:475–95.
2. Levy RM, Rosenblum S, Perrett LV. Neuroradiologic findings in AIDS: a review of 200 cases. AJNR 1986;7:833–9.
3. Post MJD, Tate LG, Quencer RM, et al. CT, MR and pathology in HIV encephalitis and meningitis. AJR 1988;151:373–80.
4. Pepito CL, Cho ES, Lemann W, et al. Neuropathology of acquired immunodeficiency syndrome (AIDS): an autopsy review. J Neuropathol Exp Neurol 1986;45:635–46.
5. Dorfman LJ. Cytomegalovirus encephalitis in adults. Neurology 1973;23:136–44.
6. Bale JF Jr. Human cytomegalovirus infection and disorders of the nervous system. Arch Neurol 1984;41:310–20.
7. Gans J de, Portegies P. Neurological complications of infection with human immunodeficiency virus Type I. Clin Neurol Neurosurg 1989;91-3:199–219.
8. Post MJD, Kursunoglu SJ, Hensley GT, et al. Cranial CT in acquired immunodeficiency syndrome: spectrum of diseases and optimal contrast enhancement technique. AJR 1985;145:929–40.
9. Whelan MA, Kricheff II, Handler M, et al. Acquired immunodeficiency snydrome: Cerebral computed tomographic manifestations. Radiology 1983;149:477–84.
10. Cohen W, Koslow M. An unusual CT presentation of cerebral toxoplasmosis. J Comput Assist Tomogr 1985;9:384–86.
11. Post MJD, Chan JC. Hensley GT, et al. Toxoplasma encephalitis in Haitian adults with acquired immunodeficiency syndrome: clinical pathologic CT correlation. AJNR 1983;140:861–8.
12. Navia BA, Petito CK, Gold JWM, et al. Cerebral toxoplasmosis complicating the acquired immune deficiency syndrome: clinical and neuropathological findings in 27 patients. Ann Neurol 1986;19:224–38.
13. Rodesch G, Parizel PM, Farber CM, et al. Nervous system manifestations and neuroradiologic findings in acquired immunodeficiency syndrome (AIDS). Neuroradiology 1989;31:33–9.
14. So YT, Beckstead JH, Davis RL. Primary central nervous system lymphoma in acquired immune deficiency syndrome: a clinical and pathological study. Ann Neurol 1986;20:566–72.
15. Poon T, Matoso I, Tcherthoff V, et al. CT features of primary cerebral lymphoma in AIDS and non-AIDS patients. J Comput Assist Tomogr 1989;13:6–9.
16. Bishburg E, Sunderam G, Reichman LB, et al. Central nervous system tuberculosis with the acquired immunodeficiency syndrome and its related complex. Ann Intern Med 1986;105:210–13.
17. Olsen WL, Longo FM, Mills CM, et al. White matter disease in AIDS: findings at MR imaging. Radiology 1988;169:445–8.
19. Navia BA, Cho ES, Petito CK, et al. The AIDS dementia complex: II. Neuropathology. Ann Neurol 1986;19:525–35.
19. Portegies P, Gans J de, Lange JMA, et al. Declining incidence of AIDS dementia complex after introduction of zidovudine treatment. Br Med J 1989;299:819–21.

20. Krupp LB, Lipton RB, Swerdlow ML, et al. Progressive multifocal leukoencephalopathy: clinical and radiographic features. Ann Neurol 1985;17:344−9.

21. Wehn SW, Heinz ER, Burger PC, et al. Dilated Virchow−Robin spaces in cryptococcal menin-gitis associated with AIDS: CT and MR findings. J Comput Assist Tomogr 1989;13:756−62.

22. Post MJD, Hensley GT, Moskowitz LB, et al. Cytomegalic inclusion virus encephalitis in patients with AIDS: clinical and pathological correlation. AJR 1986;146:1229−34.

8 Myelography in AIDS

P. A. Koster

AIDS patients frequently experience lesions of the spinal cord, including vacuolar myelopathy, viral myelitis, and (rarely) tumors. The most frequent disorder is vacuolar myelopathy, often accompanied by a peripheral neuropathy (1). The clinical picture consists of a progressive paraparesis with disturbances of sensation and urinary incontinence. In such cases, however, myelography does not reveal any abnormalities of the spinal cord, whereas in neuropathologic examination, vacuolization of the white matter of the spinal cord can be seen.

Compression of the spinal cord due to an extramedullar, localized lesion, such as metastasis of non-Hodgkin's lymphoma, epi-

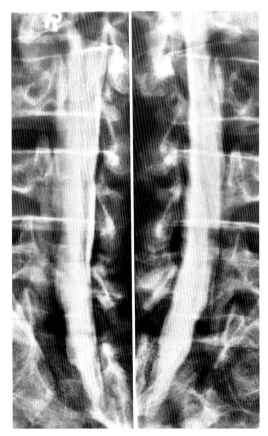

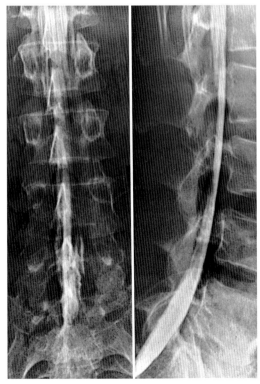

Fig. 8.1 CMV polyradiculitis in a 36-year-old man with paraparesis and problems of micturition. Myelography demonstrates extensive root adhesions in the lumbar area

Fig. 8.2 CMV polyradiculitis in a 27-year-old man. Myelography demonstrates lack of contrast due to root adhesions

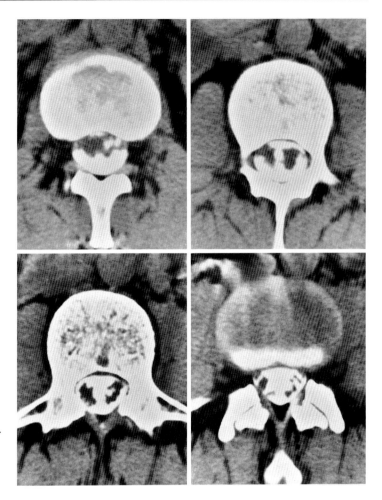

Fig. 8.3 Polyradiculitis (due to CMV) in a 40-year-old man with rapidly progressive paraparesis and urinary retention. CT following intrathecal contrast shows root adhesions in region L1–L4

dural sarcoma, or plasmocytoma, is a very rare finding in AIDS patients (2, 3). In such cases, myelography reveals the image of an epidural lesion, but further differentiation is impossible.

The peripheral nervous system in AIDS patients is frequently affected in various ways including cytomegalovirus polyradiculopathy and HIV-related peripheral neuropathy. CMV polyradiculopathy is clinically characterized by a paraparesis and disturbance of micturition, and there are descriptions in the literature of myelographic abnormalities of the caudal roots (4, 5). The latter show adhesions (Fig. 8.1) and thus form thick bundles in the dural sac, visible due to the lack of contrast (Fig. 8.2) and resembling an arachnoiditis. Using CT (after myelography), the abnormal appearance of the nerve roots in the dural sac can be visualized (Fig. 8.3).

The abnormalities mentioned have only been described in certain cases of CMV polyradiculitis; investigation of the CSF is of greater importance for the diagnosis. Myelography does not play a role in the other AIDS-related disorders of the peripheral nervous system.

Conclusion

In patients with AIDS, disorders of spinal cord, conus, cauda, and peripheral nerves are common. However, only in a very small number of cases, myelography can reveal abnormalities such as epidural lesions or (sometimes) signs of a polyradiculitis resulting from a cytomegalovirus infection, illustrating the limited value of this technique for AIDS patients.

References

1. Petito CK, Navia BA, Cho ES, et al. Vacuolar myelopathy pathologically resembling subacute combined degeneration in patients with the acquired immunodeficiency syndrome. N Engl J Med 1985; 312:874–9.
2. Snider WD, Simpson DM, Nielson S, et al. Neurological complications of acquired immune deficiency syndrome: analysis of 50 patients. Ann Neurol 1983; 403–18.
3. Federle MP. A radiologist looks at AIDS: Imaging evaluation based on symptoms complexes. Radiology 1988; 166:553–62.
4. Borgstein BJ, Koster PA, Portegies P, et al. Myelography in patients with acquired immunodeficiency syndrome, indications and results. Neuroradiology 1989; 31:326–30.
5. Eidelberg D, Sortel A, Vogel H, et al. Progressive polyradiculopathy in acquired immune deficiency syndrome. Neurology 1986; 36:912–16.

9 MRI of AIDS-related CNS Disorders

J. Valk

Introduction

Neurologic signs and symptoms are reported in 30–75% of patients with AIDS. In the majority of cases, these can be attributed to HIV encephalopathy, present as subacute encephalitis, meningitis, vacuolar myelopathy, or inflammatory demyelinating peripheral neuropathy (2, 4, 8, 9, 10).

The most frequent neurologic manifestation is subacute encephalitis, also known as AIDS encephalopathy and AIDS dementia complex. In about 30% of the cases, the neurologic manifestations are caused by opportunistic infections, such as toxoplasmosis, herpes simplex or herpes zoster encephalitis, cytomegalovirus encephalitis, *Cryptococcus neoformans* infection, and papovavirus infection. AIDS of the CNS can also manifest itself by intracranial tumors that are either not common in immunocompetent individuals or different in appearance. The best known are Kaposi's sarcoma, of which CNS manifestations have been described, and primary CNS lymphoma. Spinal cord involvement has also been reported in AIDS patients with MRI manifestation similar to that of transverse myelitis.

The Role of MRI in AIDS-related CNS Disorders

It is widely accepted that MR imaging has a higher sensitivity for detecting brain-tissue afflictions than any other imaging modality, including CT. With the increasing availability of MRI, one may expect that it will be the modality of choice for the diagnosis of subacute HIV encephalitis, opportunistic infections, and tumors of the CNS. In our experience, the use of MRI has improved the diagnosis of subacute HIV encephalitis, especially in the early phases, and the detection of toxoplasmosis infection, where in some proven cases CT was negative and MRI correlated well with histologic findings. Specificity of MRI is commonly considered to be lower than its sensitivity. This, however, is too general a statement and we will try to add a few nuances. The contributions of MRI to the diagnosis of AIDS-related CNS disorders will be dealt with under four headings:

1. MRI of subacute HIV encephalitis
2. MRI of opportunistic infections
3. MRI of neoplasms
4. MRI of other pathology of the CNS in AIDS patients

MRI of Subacute HIV Encephalitis

Postmortem studies of brains of patients with subacute HIV encephalitis show some degree of atrophy, with widened cortical sulci and dilated ventricles. The most prominent microscopic abnormalities involve the white matter and deep-seated gray matter. Subacute HIV encephalitis is characterized by parenchymal and perivascular infiltrations of lymphocytes and macrophages located both in gray and white matter. The perivascular infiltrations occur typically around capillaries and veins and are most frequently detected in the centrum semiovale, basal ganglia, and pons. The most common white matter abnormality is diffuse pallor, demonstrated by myelin staining. In the early phase of the disease, MRI already shows mild but definite signal changes in the white matter of the frontal and parietal part of the centrum semiovale, even when the macroscopic brain studies are still negative (7, 10, 11, 12; Figs. 9.**1**, 9.**2**). Microscopy then shows white matter pallor. In a much later phase, the abnormalities in the white matter become more extensive, more severe, and eventually,

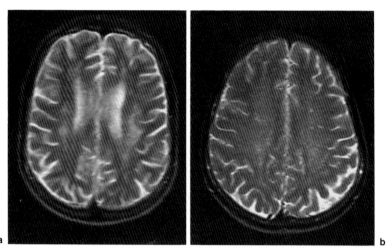

a   b

Fig. 9.**1a, b** Patient with an early phase of subacute HIV encephalitis. The T2-weighted images show diffuse, nearly symmetrical regions of high signal intensity of the white matter, in which the U fibers are spared

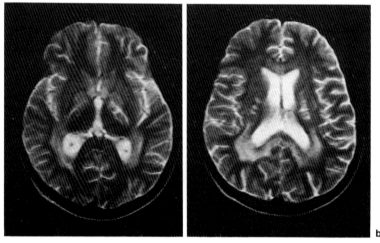

a   b

Fig. 9.**2a, b** These images show the nearly symmetrical affliction of white matter as it occurs in this more advanced case of subacute HIV encephalitis. In the slice at the level of the third ventricle (**a**) the involvement of the posterior limb of the internal capsule and the diffuse changes of the white matter bordering the lateral ventricles are clearly seen. The higher slice (**b**) also shows the symmetry of the affliction. In the early phase of the disease, the arcuate fibers are spared. Also note the involvement of genu and splenium of the corpus callosum

demonstrable on CT. This MRI pattern is specific for subacute encephalitis, which can be caused not only by AIDS but also by other afflictions such as cytomegalovirus infections. In AIDS patients, however, the pattern of mild demyelination in the frontal and parietal areas in which the U fibers are spared will nearly always represent subacute HIV encephalitis. If atrophy also exists, MRI is capable of demonstrating very well both cortical and periventricular loss of tissue, as is CT (Fig. 9.**3**).

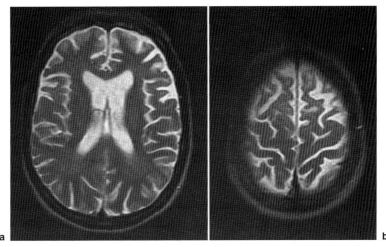

Fig. 9.**3a, b**   The most common finding in MRI of AIDS-related CNS disorders is generalized cerebral atrophy. The images demonstrate a mild widening of the ventricles and of the cortical sulci, predominantly on the left

In some cases (3%), we find other infections superimposed on this pattern of subacute encephalitis. We refer to these superinfections below. What still has to be explained is the discrepancy between the reported incidence of subacute HIV encephalitis in neuropathologic studies, as high as 50% of cases, and MRI, 5–15% of cases. Perhaps the time of the examination is of importance, as well as the possibility that the detection threshold of subacute encephalitis by MRI is still considerably higher than of histologic studies.

MRI of Opportunistic Infections

A wide variety of infections, bacterial, viral, fungal, and parasitic, occur in immunodepressed patients. Infection with toxoplasmosis occurs most frequently. Toxoplasmosis may produce cerebral abscesses, granulomas, or meningoencephalitis. On the MR images, multiple lesions, rounded and of different sizes, are usually observed as having a predilection for the basal ganglia and the corticomedullary junction, with possible spread to the gray matter. The lesions have high signal intensity on T2-weighted images, and some of the lesions show a lower signal intensity centrally, the so-called target lesions (Fig. 9.**4**). After intravenous contrast injection, most of the lesions will enhance and fill in from the outside toward the center on delayed scans. We have not seen meningeal afflictions in patients with toxoplasmosis. If multiple lesions as described above are found in an immunodepressed patient, the diagnosis of toxoplasmosis will usually be correct. The pattern is, however, not pathognomonic and similar lesions can be seen in fungal infections, tuberculosis, lymphoma, and neoplasms (5). In cases in which the initial study is performed on MRI, the monitoring of the disease should also be done on MRI and not, as is sometimes suggested, on CT. The therapeutic response of the various lesions depends on their location and complexity. The larger the lesion, and the greater the mass effect, the longer it will take for the lesion to disappear.

The second most frequent infection in immunodepressed patients is progressive multifocal leukoencephalopathy (PML), a rare demyelinating infection of the CNS caused by a papovavirus (6, 12). It is usually associated with such underlying disease as lymphoma, multiple myeloma, leukemia, sarcoidosis, tuberculosis, systemic carcinomas,

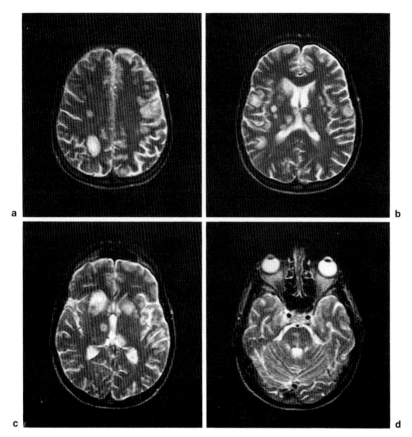

Fig. 9.**4a–d** Four slices in a seropositive patient with proven toxoplasmosis. In these T2-weighted images, multiple lesions of different size are shown, some related to the frontal horns of the ventricles and some in the basal ganglia, where on the right side a "target" lesion is seen with a lower signal intensity centrally. There are diffuse lesions in the pons

renal transplantation, AIDS, and other immunosuppressed states. It occurs mainly in adults, and there is a male preponderance of 5:3. In PML the brain shows no external abnormalities upon inspection. Yet upon sectioning, multiple grayish, granular-appearing lesions are seen in the white matter, often with loss of distinction between gray and white matter. The lesions are often asymmetric and more extensive in one hemisphere than in the other. This description concurs with the findings on MRI: asymmetrical, confluent lesions extending towards the convexity of the brain and eventually involving the gray matter (Fig. 9.**5**). A second

examination often shows the progressive nature of the disease.

Of the fungal infections, that of *cryptococcus neoformans* is the least rare in AIDS patients. It usually presents as meningitis. Affliction of the basal ganglia occurs via the Virchow–Robin spaces leading to a rather typical pattern of lesions.

Many other infections can become manifest in AIDS patients. Cytomegalovirus infections, *Escherichia coli* meningitis, tuberculosis, herpes simplex, and so on have all been described on occasion in AIDS patients. In most of these cases the MRI pattern is not pathognomonic.

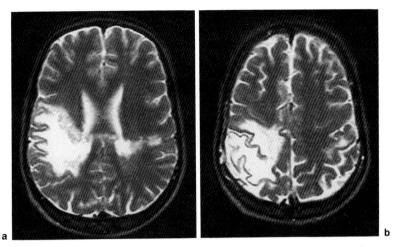

Fig. 9.**5a, b** Patient with progressive multifocal leukoencephalopathy. The lesions are asymmetrical, confluent, and extending from the corpus callosum to the subcortical white matter, eventually involving the gray matter

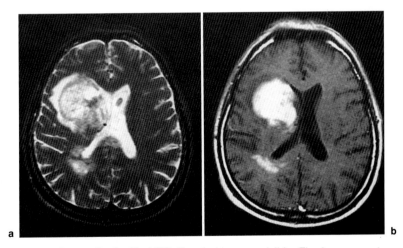

Fig. 9.**6a, b** Primary CNS lymphoma in a patient with AIDS. Two lesions are visible. The larger one is seen as a periventricular, rounded mass with inhomogeneous signal intensity and a small border of edema; the second one is located near the occipital horn, less well defined. After injection of Gd-DTPA both lesions enhance

Injection of Gd-DTPA is sometimes helpful to diagnose leptomeningeal or ventricular ependymal involvement.

MRI of Neoplasms

Primary CNS lymphomas are not uncommon in AIDS; some of them are true Burkitt's lymphomas, known to be associated with the Epstein–Barr virus. They are morphologically centered around vessels and consist of large immunoblastic cells (4). Secondary lymphomas in the CNS do occur rarely and are mostly located in the subarachnoid spaces. The primary lymphomas often present as a single lesion, though multiple lesions

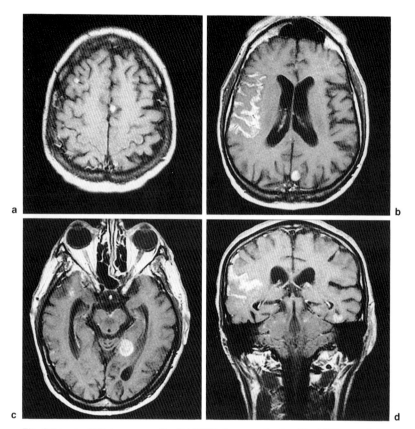

Fig. 9.**7a–d** MR images with Gd-DTPA in a patient with AIDS; mutiple, rounded lesions of different size, with enhancement and an infarction of the right middle cerebral artery also showing enhancement. Probably a combination of toxoplasmosis and cerebral infarction

have been described in AIDS patients. Most often they are located in the periventricular region, surrounded by edema, and with high signal intensity on T2-weighted MR images (Fig. 9.**6**). The centers of the lesions may show a lower intermediate signal intensity, unlike the appearance in non-AIDS patients. The lesion enhances after an injection of Gd-DTPA, possibly in a ringlike pattern. This pattern is not pathognomonic and can be mimicked by toxoplasmosis.

We have not seen cases with Kaposi's sarcoma of the CNS; this has also been reported in the literature (4).

MRI of Other Pathology of the CNS in AIDS Patients

Infarctions. In AIDS patients, infarctions occur at a younger age than usual. The lesions show the same characteristics as infarctions in a non-AIDS population (Fig. 9.**7**).

Spinal involvement. There have been reports of myelopathy and peripheral neuropathy in AIDS. In one case, spinal MRI is reported to show high signal intensity lesions on T2-weighted images, with an appearance similar to lesions seen in multiple sclerosis, idiopathic transverse myelitis, and so on (Fig. 9.**8**).

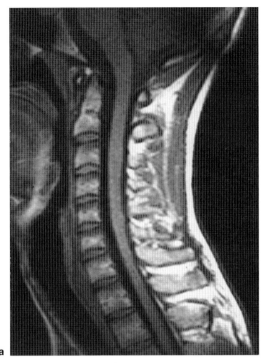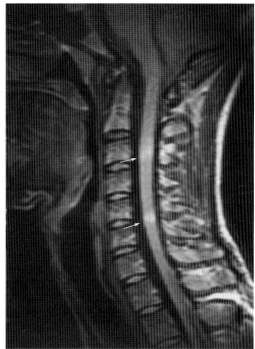

a   b

Fig. 9.**8a, b**   Patient with transverse myelitis with lesions in the cervical cord. The lesions have a high signal intensity on proton density and T2-weighted images. Similar lesions can be seen in patients with multiple sclerosis, Lyme's disease, sarcoidosis of the cord, and AIDS myelopathy

In these patients, MRI is of course the imaging modality of choice; CT and myelography would be disappointing in these cases (1, 2).

Summary

MRI is very capable of showing the lesions of CNS disorders in AIDS. Although the specificity is certainly less than the sensitivity, in quite a few cases, MRI can provide a suggestion of the underlying pathology. When MRI is used for the initial diagnosis, it should also be used for follow-up studies. A change of modality for this purpose, for example from MRI to CT, as is sometimes suggested, is inappropriate and may lead to false conclusions.

References

1. Barakos JA, Mark AS, Dillon WP, Norman D. MR imaging of acute transverse myelitis and AIDS myelopathy. J Comput Assist Tomogr 1990; 14(1):45–50.
2. Gans de J, Portegies P, Derix MMA, Troost D, Valk J, Goudsmit J. Het AIDS-dementiecomplex: een primaire infectie met humaan immunodeficiëntievirus type 1. Ned Tijdschr Geneeskd 1988; 132:1570–5.
3. Goldstick L, Mandybur TI, Bode R. Spinal cord degeneration in AIDS. Neurology 1985; 35: 103–6.
4. Gorin FA, Bale JF, Halks-Miller M, Schwartz RA. Kaposi's sarcoma metastatic to the CNS. Arch. Neurol 1985; 42:162–5.
5. Gray F, Gherardi R, Scaravilli F. The neuropathology of the acquired immune deficiency syndrome (AIDS): a review. Brain 1988; 111:245–66.
6. Kupfer MC, Zee CS, Colletti PM, Boswell WD, Rhodes R. MRI evaluation of Aids-related encephalopathy: toxoplasmosis vs. lymphoma. Magn Reson Imaging 1990; 8:51–7.

7. Mark AS, Atlas SW. Progressive multifocal leukoencephalopathy in patients with AIDS: appearance on MR images. Radiology 1989; 173:517–20.

8. Olsen WL, Longo FM, Mills CM, Norman D. White matter disease in AIDS: findings at MR imaging. Radiology 1988; 169:445–8.

9. Paz de la R, Enzmann D. Neuroradiology of acquired immunodeficiency syndrome. In: Rosenblum ML, Levy RM, Bredesen DE, eds. AIDS and the nervous system. New York: Raven Press, 1988:121–53.

10. Post MJD, Sheldon JJ, Hensley GT, et al. Central nervous system disease in acquired immunodeficiency syndrome: prospective correlation using CT, MR imaging, and pathologic studies. Radiology 1986; 158:141–8.

11. Post MJD, Tate LG, Quencer RM, et al. CT, MR, and pathology in HIV encephalitis and meningitis. AJNR 1988;9:469–76.

12. Valk J. Aids encephalopathy. In: Valk J, ed. MRI of the brain, head, neck and spine. Dordrecht: Martinus Nijhoff, 1988:264–75.

13. Valk J, vd Knaap MS. Acquired immunodeficiency syndrome. In: Valk J, vd Knaap MS, eds. Magnetic resonance of myelin, myelination, and myelin disorders. Berlin: Springer, 1989:227–40.

14. Zimmerman RA, Bilaniuk LT, Sze G. Intracranial infection. In: Brant-Zawadzki M, Norman D, eds. Magnetic resonance imaging of the central nervous system. New York: Raven Press, 1989:254–7.

10 Clinical Aspects of Pulmonary Complications in AIDS

R. P. van Steenwijk

The AIDS epidemic has brought about an important change in the type and severity of pathology the lung specialist may encounter. Of all organ systems, the respiratory tract is the one most frequently affected by infections or neoplasms which lead to the diagnosis of AIDS (1, 2). The signs and symptoms of the various pulmonary complications of AIDS strongly resemble each other. Careful analysis of history, laboratory parameters, radiodiagnostics, and pulmonary function will often lead to a limited differential diagnosis. The interpretation of radiographic abnormalities without adequate clinical data is virtually impossible. This survey will discuss the presentation of the most important infections and neoplasms.

Infections

HIV infection causes a progressive depletion of T-helper lymphocytes which play a central role in the regulation of the immune system. This leads to the extraordinary susceptibility to opportunistic infections. The degree of immunosuppression as indicated by the number of T4 cells, gives information about the probability of occurrence of a particular complication (3).

Pneumocystis carinii Pneumonia

PCP is the most frequently occurring (pulmonary) infection and responsible for considerable morbidity and mortality (2). It is seen in cases of long-term suppression of T cell–mediated immunity. Corticosteroids are very effective in evoking the infection. In addition, it is also seen after the use of cyclophosphamide, chlorambucil, and cyclosporine A. The pneumocystis infection is almost always confined to the lung. The histologic features are a foamy, cell-poor, intra-alveolar exudate, interstitial infiltration with lymphocytes, and an increase in alveolar macrophages. The cysts can be stained characteristically with Grocott–Gomori methenamine silver nitrate (Fig. 10.1). They can also be made visible with toluidine blue. The trophozoites stain with Giemsa and Gram, but are much more difficult to distinguish from background material. Compared to PCP in patients with other causes of immunosuppression, AIDS patients have a longer prodromal phase with a subacute and insidious presentation of the symptoms (4). The response to treatment is also slower, and radiologic abnormalities persist longer. Five months after treatment, the radiologic abnormalities have completely disappeared in only 43% of the patients.

Symptoms may be present for weeks or months before a diagnosis is established. The most frequently occurring are shortness of breath upon exertion (90%), fever (70%), and a nonproductive cough (50%). In addition, loss of weight, night sweats, pain in the thorax, and malaise may be present. On physical examination, the most striking findings are fever and tachypnea. Laboratory investigation reveals a normal leukocyte count with lymphopenia. The number of T4 cells is usually less than 0.2×10^9/L. Arterial blood gas analysis can reveal hypoxemia and hypocapnea of considerable severity (2). Pulmonary function tests show a restrictive disorder and a decreased CO diffusing capacity. The gallium-67 scintigraphy is abnormal in 93% of cases, even when the X-ray of the chest is normal. A normal gallium scan in particular has a high negative predictive value (7, 8).

The most common radiographic presentation is a diffuse, bilateral interstitial and/or alveolar infiltrate with a ground-glass

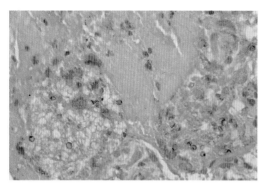

Fig. 10.**1** *Pneumocystis carinii* pneumonia with fibrosis (silver methenamine stain)

appearance. In 6–23% of the patients, the chest radiograph is normal or only slightly abnormal. Lobar or segmental infiltrates are also one of the initial presentations. Should PCP arise in spite of the prophylactic inhalation of pentamidine, the abnormalities are often located in the upper regions. Pleural fluid is an uncommon finding in PCP.

The diagnosis is established by demonstrating the pneumocysts. Bronchoscopy with transbronchial peripheral lung biopsy and bronchoalveolar lavage (BAL) has a sensitivity up to 100%. Pneumocysts can also be demonstrated in induced sputum. PCP is preferentially treated with high doses of co-trimoxazole. Provided it is treated in time, the prognosis is good. If respiratory insufficiency makes artificial respiration necessary, the mortality is high (80–90%; 2). After treatment, lifelong maintenance therapy is essential. Maintenance therapy with co-trimoxazole is effective and generally well tolerated. Some patients have adverse reactions to co-trimoxazole. An alternative prophylactic is inhalation of aerosolized pentamidine which lacks all the adverse reactions of the intramuscular or intravenous route. This prophylactic is, however, less efficacious, as appears from a relapse rate for PCP of approximately 13%.

Mycobacterial Infections

Mycobacterium tuberculosis

Extrapulmonary human tuberculosis (TBC) in cases of HIV seropositivity is a new criterion for AIDS as defined by the Centers for Disease Control (10). The incidence of active TBC in HIV-infected individuals is a reflection of the prevalence of TBC infection in the population from which the HIV-seropositive group is derived (11). The HIV infection with reduced T-cell immunity leads to rapid dissemination of the mycobacterial infection and little or no granulomatous inflammation. The tuberculin skin test is false negative in a large percentage of patients, mostly those with more advanced immunodeficiency. The clinical presentation of TBC is atypical: weight loss, fever, malaise and fatigue, and cough. Although most patients will have a reactivation of TBC, the disturbed immune response leads to a radiographic pattern resembling primary TBC: hilar or mediastinal lymphadenopathy, with or without noncavitating pulmonary infiltrates. Infiltrates in the inferior lobes and diffuse or miliary infiltrates also appear. A high index of suspicion for TBC and an aggressive diagnostic approach is needed to avoid missing a highly treatable and contagious disease. The radiologic differential diagnosis of lymphadenopathy includes, in addition to TBC, cryptococcosis, lymphoma, and Kaposi's sarcoma. The diagnosis is established by demonstrating acid-fast bacilli in (induced) sputum, BAL fluid, or lung biopsy. A good impression of the extent of the TBC can be obtained using a gallium scan, ultrasound and CT. Treatment involves three or four anti-TBC drugs, as usual, and takes 9 months. The reaction to chemotherapy both clinically and radiologically is amazingly swift.

Nontuberculous Mycobacterial Infections

Mycobacterium avium–intracellulare complex (MAI) is the mycobacterium most frequently isolated in AIDS (12). The exact prevalence of MAI is not known because of the

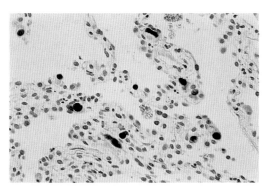

Fig. 10.2   CMV (immune peroxidase stain)

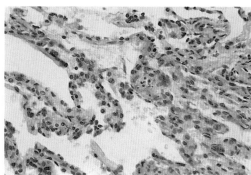

Fig. 10.3   Cryptococcus (Giemsa stain)

insidiousness of the disease and the relatively late presentation compared to other HIV-related infections. The clinical presentation is again extremely unspecific and consists mainly of general symptoms (fever, anorexia). Lymphadenopathy or hepatosplenomegaly is sometimes found. Pulmonary symptomatology is unusual. The diagnosis is made by culturing the microorganism from the blood, stools, BAL, or lung biopsy. Treatment of MAI is largely symptomatic.

Cytomegalovirus Infection

Cytomegalovirus (CMV) pneumonitis is a characteristic syndrome and a life-threatening disease in the immunocompromised, especially in transplant patients. In AIDS patients, however, CMV is of less importance as a pulmonary pathogen. CMV can be cultured from the BAL fluid in about 35% of patients (2; Fig. 10.2). Cytopathologic changes as a result of CMV are seen less often. Unequivocal data about CMV as a sole pathogenic cause of pneumonitis are scarce. When strict criteria are used for the diagnosis of CMV pneumonitis in AIDS as far as clinical data, histopathologic changes, and culture are concerned, one can expect antiviral therapy to have an effect (13).

Bacterial Infections

Because of a reduced T-cell induction of B-cell function, bacterial pneumonitis occurs more often in AIDS (12). Infections with *Streptococcus pneumoniae* and *Hemophilus influenzae* are seen with increased frequency. *H. influenzae* can present as a diffuse infiltrate in the lung which strongly resembles PCP (14, 15). *Legionella* and *Nocardia* are encountered less often than one might expect on the basis of the immune deficiency and epidemiology.

Fungi

Following *Candida albicans* and PCP, the most frequently occurring opportunistic infection is caused by *Cryptococcus neoformans* (16). Although the majority of patients (up to 85%) present with meningitis, 5% present with primary pulmonary disease. A pulmonary localization can be demonstrated in more than half the patients with cryptococcal meningitis (17). Clinically, cryptococcal pneumonia presents with sometimes productive cough, fever, and shortness of breath. Cryptococcal antigen can be demonstrated serologically. A false-negative antigen titer is, however, found in extraneural cryptococcosis (17). The chest X-ray reveals localized or diffuse infiltrates. Pleural fluid may also be present. The pulmonary localization of cryptococci is demonstrated by means of bronchoscopy with BAL (Fig. 10.3). *Histoplasma capsulatum* and coccidioidomycosis are mainly found in endemic regions. Neither *Aspergillus* nor *Candida* is regarded as an important lung pathogen in AIDS.

Neoplasm

Kaposi's sarcoma

Kaposi's sarcoma (KS) occurs in about 20% of patients with AIDS. In a later phase of sarcomal spread, the visceral organs are also affected. If localized in the lung, symptoms such as cough, dyspnea, hemoptysis, and fever can appear. Respiratory insufficiency is the ultimate result. As KS is a slowly progressive disease compared to the infections frequently seen in AIDS, the radiologic abnormalities arise gradually. These are characterized by bilateral infiltrates with an interstitial, alveolar, or nodular pattern (18). Obstruction infiltrates can occur in the case of bronchial obstruction. Pleural effusions are frequently seen in pulmonary KS, probably as a result of lymph node involvement with lymph flow obstruction. The presence of pulmonary KS can be confined by bronchoscopy when the typical lesions are visualized. Bronchial biopsies of these lesions generally do not establish the diagnosis because of the deep submucosal localization of the tumor. On occasion, KS can be demonstrated in peripheral transbronchial biopsies. Tumor regression can be achieved with chemotherapy or radiotherapy.

Lymphoma

Non-Hodgkin's lymphoma is one of the diagnostic criteria for AIDS if HIV positivity has been proved. The clinical presentation is not different from that of HIV-negative patients. One should think of lymphoma particularly if there is mediastinal and hilar enlargement of lymph nodes and in the case of pleural fluid. The prognosis is poor.

Lymphocytic Interstitial Pneumonitis (LIP)

LIP is a lymphocytic infiltration of the lung with no indications of vasculitis. There is possibly a relationship with the Epstein–Barr virus, although there is also speculation that the HIV infection itself plays a role in the occurrence of LIP (19).

LIP occurs mainly in children with AIDS. The most important symptoms are shortness of breath, pulmonary infiltrates, and growth retardation. Also in adults the appearance resembles the more frequently occurring infections such as PCP. This makes invasive diagnostic procedures necessary. The prognosis is reasonable. Spontaneous regression does occur. There is also a good response to corticosteroids.

References

1. Klatt EC. Diagnostic findings in patients with the acquired immunodeficiency syndrome (AIDS). J AIDS 1988;1:459–65.
2. Murray JF, Felton CP, Garay SM. Pulmonary complications of the acquired immunodeficiency syndrome: report of a national heart, lung and blood institute workshop. N Engl J Med 1984;310:1682–8.
3. Moss AR, Bacchetti P, Osmond D, et al. Seropositivity for HIV and the development of AIDS or AIDS-related conditions: three year follow-up of the San Francisco General Hospital cohort. Br Med J 1988;296:745–50.
4. Kovacs JA, Hiemenz JW, Macher AM, et al. *Pneumocystis carinii* pneumonia: a comparison between patients with the immunodeficiency syndrome and patients with other immunodeficiencies. Ann Intern Med 1984; 100:663–71.
5. DeLorenzo LJ, Huang CT, Maguire GP, et al. Roentgenographic patterns of *Pneumocystis carinii* pneumonia in 104 patients with AIDS. Chest 1987;91:323.
6. Macfarlane JT, Finch RG. *Pneumocystis carinii* pneumonia. Thorax 1985;40:561–70.
7. Reinders Folmer SCC, Danner SA, Bakker AJ, et al. Gallium-67 longscintigraphy in patients with the acquired immunodeficiency syndrome. Eur J Respir Dis 1986;68:313–18.
8. Barron TF, Birnbaum NS, Shane LB, et al. *Pneumocystis carinii* pneumonia studied by gallium-67 scanning. Radiology 1985;154:791.
9. Centers of Disease Control. Guidelines for prophylaxis against *Pneumocystis carinii* pneumonia for persons infected with human immunodeficiency virus. JAMA 1989; 262:335–9.
10. Centers for Disease Control. Revision of the CDC surveillance case definition for acquired immunodeficiency syndrome. MMWR 1987 (suppl) 36:3s–15s.

11. Chaisson RE, Schecter GF, Theuer CP, et al. Tuberculosis in patients with the acquired immunodeficiency syndrome: clinical features, response to therapy and survival. Am Rev Respir Dis 1987;136:570–4.
12. Fauci AS. Acquired immunodeficiency syndrome: Epidemiologic, clinical, immunologic and therapeutic considerations. Ann Intern Med 1984;110:92–106.
13. Jacobson MA, Mills J. Cytomegalovirus infection. In: White DA, Stover DE, eds. Pulmonary effects of AIDS. Clin Chest Med 1988;9:443–8.
14. Armstrong D, Gold JWM, Dryjanski J, et al. Treatment of infections in patients with the acquired immunodeficiency syndrome. Ann Intern Med 1985;103:738–43.
15. Polsky B, Gold JWM, Whimbey E, et al. Bacterial pneumonia in patients with the acquired immunodeficiency syndrome. Ann Intern Med 1986;104:38–41.
16. Zuger A, Louie E, Holzman RS, et al. Cryptococcal disease in patients with the acquired immunodeficiency syndrome. Ann Intern Med 1986;104:234.
17. Kovacs JA, Kovacs AA, Polis M, et al. Cryptococcosis in the acquired immunodeficiency syndrome. Ann Intern Med 1985;103:533–8.
18. Kaplan LD, Hopewell PC, Jaffe H, Goodman PC, Bottles K, Volberding PA. Kaposi's sarcoma involving the lung in patients with the acquired immunodeficiency syndrome. J AIDS 1988;1:23–30.
19. Teirstein AS, Rosen MJ. Lymphocytic interstitial pneumonitis. In: White DA, Stover DE, eds. Pulmonary effects of AIDS. Clin Chest Med 1988;9:467–71.

11 Radiology of Lung Disorders in AIDS: Conventional Chest X-ray and Computed Tomography

J. A. Dol, F. H. Barneveld Binkhuysen

Introduction

Lung disorders are a frequent occurrence in AIDS. Abnormalities one can encounter on conventional chest X-ray and in computed tomography (CT) of the chest in patients with AIDS are classified in this chapter into these categories: infections, tumors, and other disorders.

Infections

Pneumocystis carinii

The appearance of abnormalities on the chest X-ray in a case of *Pneumocystis carinii* pneumonia (PCP) lags behind the clinical appearance. An active PCP may well be accompanied by a normal chest X-ray in about 10% of patients (1, 2, 3, 4). High-resolution CT (HRCT) can demonstrate abnormalities in this situation (5, 6). The classic image of PCP on the chest X-ray is a bilateral perihilar or basal fine interstitial pattern without pleural fluid and without hilar or mediastinal abnormalities (Fig. 11.1). This pattern often adopts a so-called ground-glass appearance.

Although the abnormalities on the chest X-ray are initially interstitial in nature, histopathologic examination reveals a predominant filling of the alveoli with inflammatory exudate early in the course of the disease. As the infection progresses, signs of air-space disease in the form of scattered alveolar consolidations also appear on the chest X-ray. The first abnormal manifestation of PCP in CT is a symmetrical ground-glass appearance of the lung parenchyma, while the lung periphery may well be spared (Fig. 11.2).

Later in the course of the disease, asymmetrically scattered alveolar consolidations can be seen; there is often a mosaic pattern of affected and unaffected (sub)-

segments and sometimes a predominantly reticular pattern caused by thickening of interlobular and/or intralobular interstitial tissue. Just like the chest X-ray, CT seldom demonstrates intrathoracic lymphadenopathy or pleural fluid (Fig. 11.3).

The final stage of PCP is a life-threatening respiratory insufficiency which can be associated with ARDS. The concomitant radiologic abnormalities cannot be distinguished from those of other causes of ARDS (7).

Sometimes atypical images are seen in PCP, as summarized in Table 11.1 (1, 3, 4, 8, 9, 10, 11, 12, 13).

Cavities in PCP are almost always thin-walled and usually occur in the upper lobes (irrespective of the distribution of other abnormalities; 13, 14, 15). These pneumatoceles may arise early or late in the course of the disease and can persist after the pneumonia has disappeared (Fig. 11.4). A complication of PCP associated with the presence of pneumatoceles is spontaneous pneumothorax. Abnormalities which are confined to the upper regions occur more often in patients who use pentamidine inhalation prophylaxis (11, 12).

Usually there is a definite improvement in the chest X-ray appearance 2 weeks after initiating antibiotic therapy, followed by normalization. The radiologic abnormalities persist in some patients, however, despite the fact that the pneumonia seems to have been cured from a clinical and microbiological point of view. These usually take the form of bilateral reticular or reticulonodular patterns on the chest X-ray. HRCT then reveals a corresponding interstitial pattern. Histopathologically, these patients seem to have interstitial fibrosis (16). The occurrence of this disorder is not linked to previous oxygen administra-

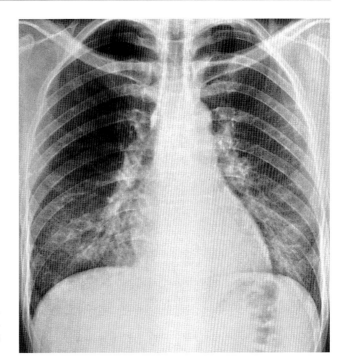

Fig. 11.**1** *Pneumocystis carinii* pneumonia. The chest X-ray shows reticular shadowing bilaterally in the
inferior regions

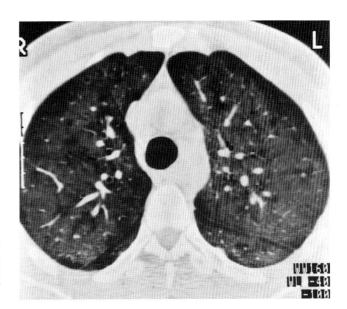

Fig. 11.**2** *Pneumocystis carinii* pneumonia. HRCT displays the diffuse,
ground-glass appearance of the lung
parenchyma; the periphery is relatively unaffected

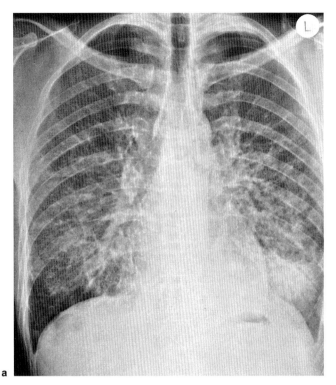

a

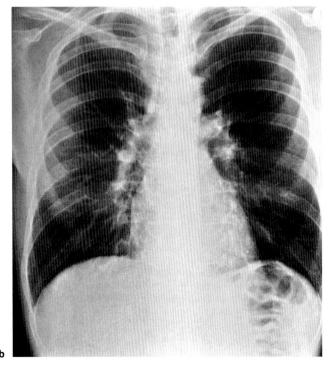

b

Fig. 11.**3** *Pneumocystis carinii* pneumonia. **a** The chest X-ray shows diffuse reticular shadowing and also focal consolidation and pleural fluid on the left

b The same patient, a few weeks later, during treatment for PCP. The chest X-ray shows regression of the abnormalities, including the pleural fluid

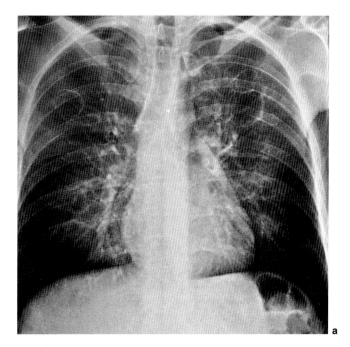

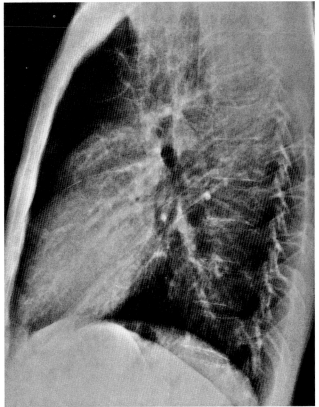

Fig. 11.**4**   Pneumatoceles in PCP. In addition to reticular abnormalities, the PA (**a**) and lateral (**b**) chest X-rays show thin-walled cavities in both upper lobes

Table 11.1   Atypical thorax images in PCP and their frequency as reported in the literature

Abnormalities confined to the upper lobes
   (incidental)
Unilateral abnormalities (0–6%)
Cavity formation (0–13%)
Solitary/multiple nodules (incidental)
Intrathoracic lymph gland enlargement (0–5%)
Pleural fluid (0–2%)
Spontaneous pneumothorax (1–6%)

tion or other therapy. If PCP recurs, a mixed image emerges of fibrosis and infection. With regard to interpretation in this situation, it is very important to compare the most recent images with previous ones.

Mycobacterium tuberculosis

Infection of the lung with *Mycobacterium tuberculosis* occurs more often in AIDS patients than in the general population. Just as in non-AIDS patients, several patterns of disease can be distinguished. A sign of primary tuberculosis is enlargement of hilar and/or mediastinal lymph glands, in some cases accompanied by pulmonary infiltration. Infiltration does not seem to show any preference for a particular region of the lung. The postprimary form manifests as infiltrative abnormalities with a preference for the upper lobe and the superior segment of the lower lobe, not usually accompanied by lymphadenopathy. A third form is miliary tuberculosis in which hematogenous dissemination of tubercle bacilli produces a diffuse, fine, nodular pattern on chest X-ray. In the majority of adult tuberculosis patients who do not have AIDS, the postprimary form of pulmonary tuberculosis is seen; the primary infection and miliary tuberculosis occur relatively seldom in this group. AIDS patients with tuberculosis do usually have the primary form (± 60%), while miliary tuberculosis is also seen more often (± 15%) than in non-AIDS patients (Figs. 11.5, 11.6; 17, 18). Pulmonary cavities are rare in cases of AIDS and more common in non-AIDS patients. Pleural fluid is present sometimes, both in AIDS and in non-AIDS

patients. In cases of pulmonary tuberculosis in non-AIDS patients, a chest X-ray with no abnormalities is rarely seen. This occurs in ± 5% of AIDS patients.

If conventional chest X-rays do not provide sufficient information, CT can provide further information concerning the localization and extent of abnormalities of the lung parenchyma and of possible lymphadenopathy.

Atypical Mycobacteria

Tuberculosis is generally seen early in the course of AIDS and may be the first manifestation. On the other hand, infection with atypical mycobacteria occurs late in ± 20% of the patients with AIDS (2). The most frequently encountered atypical mycobacterium is *Mycobacterium avium–intracellulare* (MAI). *Mycobacterium kansasii* is seen less often. In the non-immunodeficient host, MAI infection is a primary pulmonary process which expresses itself radiologically as patchy infiltrates or nodules with a tendency to form cavities and a preference for the superior lobes. In contrast, in AIDS patients MAI is almost always a disseminated process, not always affecting the lung (anymore), although it is assumed that this is the point of entry. Thus, abnormalities are rarely seen on the chest X-ray. If the lung is affected, diffuse or localized patchy infiltrates or nodules with or without indications of intrathoracic lymphadenopathy can be seen (Figs. 11.7, 11.8). This latter disorder can also occur without pulmonary abnormalities (19, 20, 21, 22). One might expect a similar spectrum of findings in *Mycobacterium kansasii* infections. Because of the late occurrence of infection with this atypical mycobacterium, the image is usually mixed because of the simultaneous presence of other pathogens.

Fungi

Fungal infections in AIDS are usually disseminated. Fungal pneumonia occurs in less than 5% of AIDS patients (2). *Cryptococcus*

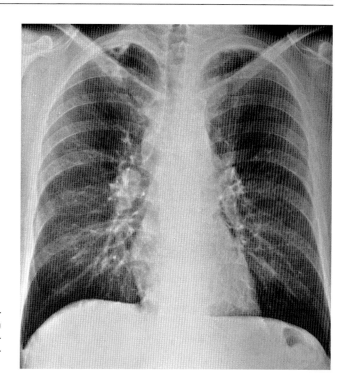

Fig. 11.**5** Tuberculosis. The chest X-ray displays gland enlargement in the right hilar region and tracheo-bronchially, and a small cavity-forming lesion in the right apex

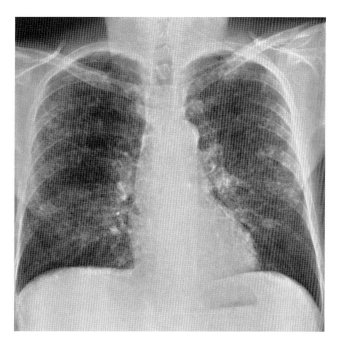

Fig. 11.**6** Miliary tuberculosis. The chest X-ray shows a diffuse, fine, nodular pattern

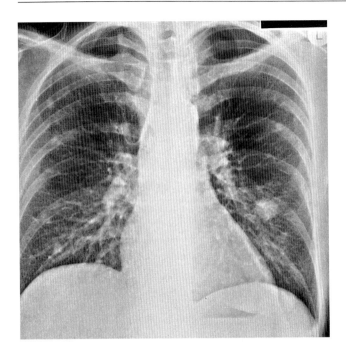

Fig. 11.**7** MAI infection. Bilaterally distributed nodules are visible on the chest X-ray

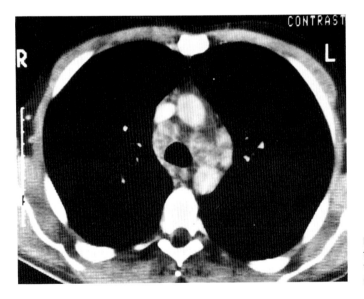

Fig. 11.**8** MAI infection. CT at the level of the aortopulmonary window shows mediastinal lymph gland enlargement

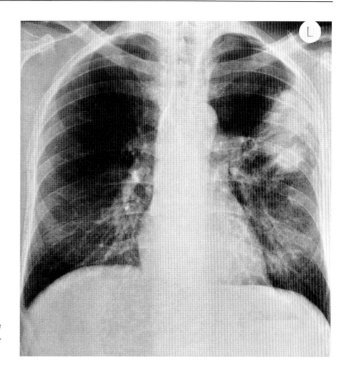

Fig. 11.**9** *Nocardia* pneumonia. The chest X-ray shows an area of consolidation in the left upper lobe

neoformans is the most common pathogenic fungus in AIDS. Other fungi, such as *Histoplasma capsulatum, Candida albicans, Aspergillus fumigatus, Nocardia asteroides*, and *Coccidioides immites* are found less often. In cryptococcal pneumonia, there is a large diversity of radiologic expression: a solitary nodule or multiple nodules with or without cavities, a miliary pattern, segmental consolidation, and bilaterally scattered, patchy infiltrates may be encountered. Intrathoracic lymphadenopathy is often (± 80%) present, sometimes with normal lung parenchyma. Pleural fluid is sometimes present in cryptococcal pneumonia (23, 24, 25). In AIDS patients, pneumococcal pneumonia often occurs together with a cryptococcal meningitis. Radiologically, other fungi can present in many ways; two of these produce striking images on the chest X-ray (2, 26). Nocardiosis usually appears together with a unilateral segmental or lobar consolidation, often with cavity formation (Fig. 11.**9**). Coccidioidomycosis usually expresses itself as solitary or multiple cavity-forming lesions which often have a thin wall (2).

Viruses

Viral pneumonia in AIDS is predominantly caused by members of the herpes group: cytomegalovirus (CMV), herpes simplex virus (HSV), and varicella-zoster virus (VZV; 27). CMV is the most frequently isolated cause of viral pneumonia in AIDS patients. In most cases, chest X-ray demonstrates bilateral interstitial abnormalities which cannot be distinguished from the classic pattern of PCP. A nodular (including miliary) pattern or asymmetrically scattered alveolar opacities with a preference for central and lower regions are sometimes observed (28). Spontaneous pneumothorax and pneumomediastinum are reported as a frequent complication of severe CMV pneumonia in non-AIDS patients with compromised immunity. It seems probable that this also applies in cases of AIDS-related CMV.

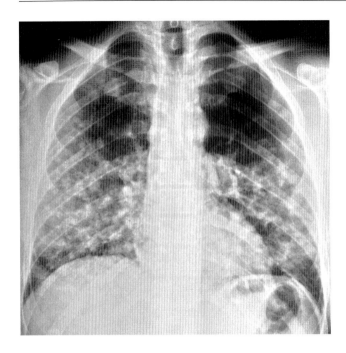

Fig. 11.**10**   Varicella-zoster viral pneumonia. The chest X-ray shows scattered focal consolidations

HSV pneumonia can manifest with a bilateral interstitial pattern just as in PCP and CMV, but (scattered) focal alveolar abnormalities occur just as often (29).

VZV pneumonia usually appears as bilaterally scattered round alveolar opacities, sometimes also described as nodular, with a tendency to coalesce (Fig. 11.**10**).

All herpesvirus pneumonias can be accompanied by a normal chest image; pleural fluid and intrathoracic lymphadenopathy are relatively rare.

Bacteria

Streptococcus pneumoniae and *Hemophilus influenzae* are among the most frequently found bacterial lung infections in AIDS, as well as *Legionella pneumoniae*. Bacterial pneumonia can manifest in AIDS patients with a chest image of unilateral or bilateral lobar consolidation. In AIDS (and other immune deficiencies), often a pattern of scattered, nonlobar consolidations may be seen (30, 31).

The development of these abnormalities is probably associated with the degree of immune disturbance. Cavity formation does occur, particularly in infections caused by staphylococci and anaerobes. Multiple lung abscesses as a result of septic emboli from intravenous drug abuse may occur in both AIDS and non-AIDS patients. The presence of pleural fluid is not unusual, particularly in infections with anaerobes, gram-negatives, staphylococci, and streptococci. In such cases, one should consider the possibility of empyema. Also in cases of AIDS, intrathoracic lymph gland enlargement does not usually occur in bacterial infections of the lung.

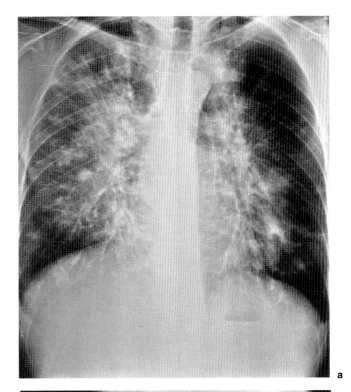

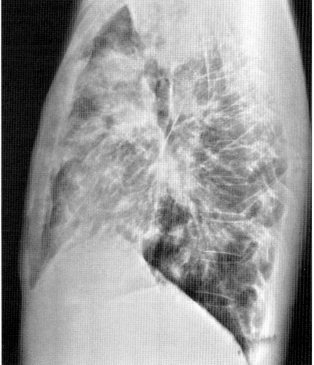

Fig. 11.**11**   Pulmonary Kaposi's sarcoma. The PA (**a**) and lateral (**b**) chest X-rays show bilateral, radiating, coarse reticular shadowing in the perihilar region and scattered round opacities

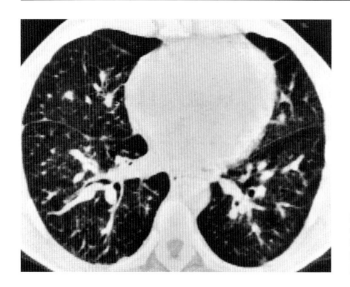

Fig. 11.**12** Pulmonary Kaposi's sarcoma. HRCT at the level of influx of the lower pulmonary veins. Thickening of fissures, interlobular septa, and peribronchovascular interstitium

Tumors

Kaposi's Sarcoma

KS in AIDS is a multicentric process which in ± 25% of cases leads to a clinically significant (pleuro)pulmonary affection. Pulmonary KS is preceded in 95% of the patients by KS lesions of skin and mucous membranes (32, 35). The chest image can display the following abnormalities (33, 34, 36):

- Bilateral reticular nodular opacities often localized in the perihilar region (Fig. 11.**11**)
- Bilaterally scattered, mostly round opacities whose delineation varies in definition
- Unilateral abnormalities (< 10%)
- Pleural fluid, mostly bilateral, often in large amounts (< 40%)
- Intrathoracic lymphadenopathy (±30%)

The interstitial abnormalities are in general coarser in nature than those which are seen in PCP; sometimes there is a fine interstitial pattern that could fit either PCP or CMV pneumonia equally well.

In CT of the chest, there is often noticeable thickening of the peribronchovascular interstitium, radiating from the perihilar region.

Endotracheal or endobronchial localizations may also be present (Fig. 11.**12**).

The lung abnormalities progress relatively slowly (over a number of months), and in the case of focal involvement, the boundary becomes increasingly unclear (Fig. 11.**13**). Atelectasis can occur because of obstruction of a bronchus.

Malignant Lymphoma

The incidence of AIDS-related lymphomas (ARL) in cases of AIDS is greater than that of malignant lymphoma in the rest of the population. Non-Hodgkin's lymphoma is the most frequently occurring ARL. Thoracic organs are relatively rarely affected in ARL (< 10%).

If the thorax is involved in the process, lymphadenopathy, pleural fluid, and intrapulmonary abnormalities can arise. In the latter case, the aspect of the lung can display a unilateral or bilateral reticular and/or nodular pattern, but a solitary mass can also appear. Pulmonary abnormalities, lymphadenopathy, and pleural fluid can each arise in isolation, but also in combination (2, 5, 34).

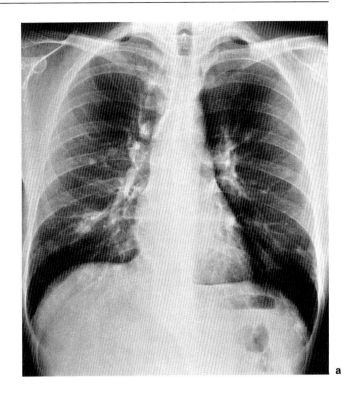

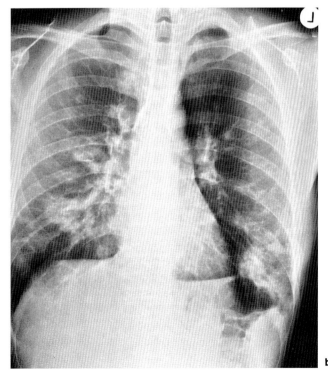

Fig. 11.**13** Pulmonary Kaposi's sarcoma. **a** The chest X-ray shows bilaterally scattered focal opacities. **b** The same patient, 3 months later. The abnormalities are larger and less sharply defined

Other Disorders

Lymphocytic Interstitial Pneumonitis

LIP is the lung disorder which occurs most frequently in children with AIDS. It is, however, also found in adults. In half of the cases, the chest X-ray is normal. If the chest X-ray displays abnormalities, these usually consist of a bilateral interstitial pattern in accordance with the classic image of PCP. Considerable development of the abnormalities and alveolar consolidations, such as those which occur in an advanced PCP, are rare in LIP. The presence of pleural fluid is unusual in LIP. Intrathoracic lymphadenopathy has not been reported in LIP (2, 37, 38).

Hypersensitivity Reactions

Allergic reactions to drugs do occur in AIDS patients, but there is usually a lack of radiologically recognizable pulmonary abnormalities. Noncardiogenic lung edema and a diffuse interstitial reticular or nodular pattern may occur. Intrathoracic lymphadenopathy and pleural fluid are sometimes seen as a result of hypersensitivity (39).

Bullous Changes

Bullous changes of the lung are seen more often in AIDS patients and at a younger age than in the general population. The bullae are mainly located in the lung periphery (in particular in the apex), in contrast to the pneumatoceles in PCP, which are found distributed in the lung parenchyma (largely in the upper lobes).

Pneumatoceles usually disappear when the pneumonia has been cured, but they can persist for a long time and cannot always be distinguished from bullae (3, 13, 15).

CT, in particular HRCT, is more sensitive than chest X-rays for tracing bullae, and their distribution can also be better determined with CT. In a recent series, using CT, bullous abnormalities were found in ± 40% of the AIDS patients with pulmonary symptoms (14).

(Peri)cardial abnormalities

Pericardial fluid in AIDS is sometimes seen as a result of tuberculosis and, incidentally, in pericardial or epicardial localizations of Kaposi's sarcoma. Cardiogenic lung edema and pleural fluid, which can, for instance, occur in the context of an AIDS-related cardiomyopathy (40), should not be confused with a progression of the infectious abnormalities in the case of pre-existent infection.

Discussion

No single radiologic finding or combination of findings is pathognomonic for a particular pathogen. Indications for radiologic investigation of the thorax include:

1. Correlation of the radiologic manifestations with the clinical picture. If the chest X-ray is unusual for the clinically determined diagnosis (established, e.g., by means of bronchoscopy or bronchoalveolar lavage), there may be additional causes which were not suspected
2. Support of bronchoscopy or bronchoalveolar lavage (BAL) on the basis of indications. If there is clinical suspicion of PCP, there is a tendency to instigate empirical treatment aimed at *Pneumocystis carinii* without invasive diagnostics (41, 42, 43, 44). If the chest X-ray or CT displays an unusual image for PCP, this can be a reason for carrying out bronchoscopy or BAL.
3. Demonstration of complications
4. As a parameter to measure the effect of treatment
5. Determination of the distribution of abnormalities
6. Determination of the precise localization of an abnormality

The following observations are important:

1. Intrathoracic adenopathy is very uncommon in PCP and in viral and bacterial infections. It is usually the result of tuberculosis, fungal infections, Kaposi's sarcoma, or malignant lymphoma.

2. Presence of pleural fluid is, certainly in large amounts, unusual in PCP and in viral infections, and occurs as a result of Kaposi's sarcoma, lymphoma, and bacterial and mycobacterial infections.

3. Thick-walled cavities are unusual in PCP, viral infections, Kaposi's sarcoma, and lymphoma. These are seen most often in cases of fungal and bacterial infections. Cavity formation does occur in mycobacterial infections, but is not usually present in tuberculosis in AIDS.

4. Thin-walled cavity formation occurs as a result of PCP (pneumatoceles), sometimes in fungal infections (coccidioidomycosis) and can also be due to bullae.

5. A solitary nodule is a most unusual manifestation of PCP and viral and bacterial infections; more likely causes are Kaposi's sarcoma, lymphoma, fungi, and mycobacteria. A diagnosis of bronchial carcinoma can also be considered, partly because an increased occurrence of this disorder is reported in AIDS.

6. Multiple nodules are unusual in PCP and bacterial infections and are mainly encountered in Kaposi's sarcoma and in cases of viral, mycobacterial, and fungal infection. The miliary pattern is mainly due to typical and atypical mycobacteria and fungi (in particular, *Cryptococcus* and *Histoplasma*).

7. Unilobar consolidation is unusual in infection with *Pneumocystis carinii*, virus, mycobacteria, and with Kaposi's sarcoma and lymphoma. It is usually the result of bacteria or fungi (especially *Nocardia*).

CT can contribute to the diagnosis. On the one hand this is possible because the presence of significant pathology can be demonstrated with a greater sensitivity than with, for example, the chest X-ray, on the other hand because it provides more accurate information about the localization of the abnormalities to be subjected to biopsy.

– Pathological lymph glands can be detected and their localization established, making a targeted biopsy possible.

– Pulmonary abnormalities whose exact position is not clear on the chest X-ray can be localized, thus aiding biopsy. For example, characteristics such as cavity formation and distribution of the abnormalities can be revealed with certainty. This can be of assistance in reaching a probable diagnosis, e.g., if a bronchoscopic diagnosis cannot be obtained.

– Pleural abnormalities can be distinguished more easily from pulmonary lesions than on the chest X-ray.

Conclusion

In spite of the fact that the radiologic image is not specific for most diseases which occur in the chest in AIDS patients, both conventional investigation as well as the (supplementary) HRCT are important for the diagnosis and therapy of this patient population. The chest X-ray plays an important part in drawing attention to unusual images indicating pathology which might or might not be expected. In addition, complications can be ascertained and the therapeutic result followed. If necessary, CT and in particular the high sensitivity of high-resolution CT can provide initial as well as additional information about the presence of abnormalities and/or their characterization and localization.

References

1. Suster B, Akerman M, Orenstein M, Wax MR. Pulmonary manifestations of AIDS: review of 106 episodes. Radiology 1986; 161:93–97.
2. Naidich DP, Garay SM, Leitman BS, McCanley DI. Radiographic manifestations of pulmonary disease in the acquired immunodeficiency syndrome (AIDS). Semin Roentgenol vol 22, no 1, 1987:14–30.
3. Lorenzo LJ, Huang CT, Stone DJ. Roentgenographic patterns of *Pneumocystis carinii* pneumonia in 104 patients with AIDS. Chest 1987;91(3):323–7.
4. Cohen BA, Pomeranz S, Rabinowitz JG, et al. Pulmonary complications of AIDS: radiologic features. AJR 1984;143:115–22.

5. Kuhlman JE, Fishman EK, Hruban RH, et al. Diseases of the chest in AIDS: CT diagnosis. Radiographics 1989, vol 9, no. 5:827–57.

6. Kuhlman JE, Kavuru M, Fishman EK, Siegelman SS. *Pneumocystis carinii* pneumonia: spectrum of parenchymal CT findings. Radiology 1990;175:711–14.

7. Maxfield RA, Sorkin B, Fazzini EP, et al. Respiratory failure in patients with acquired immunodeficiency syndrome and *Pneumocystis carinii* pneumonia. Crit Care Med 1986; 14(5):443–9.

8. Barrio JL, Suarez M, Rodriguez JL, et al. *Pneumocystis carinii* pneumonia presenting as cavitating and non cavitating solitary pulmonary nodules in patients with the acquired immunodeficiency syndrome. Am Rev Respir Dis 1986; 134:1094–6.

9. Klein JS, Warnock M, Webb WR, Gamsu G. Cavitating and noncavitating granulomas in AIDS patients in pneumocystis pneumonitis. AJR 1989;152:753–4.

10. Goodman PC, Daley C, Minagi H. Spontaneous pneumothorax in AIDS patients with *Pneumocystis carinii* pneumonia. AJR 1986; 147:29–31.

11. Bradburne RM, Ettensohn DB, Opal SM, McCool FD. Relapse of *Pneumocystis carinii* pneumonia in the upper lobes during aerosol pentamidine prophylaxis. Thorax 1989;44:591–3.

12. Chaffey MH, Klein JS, Gamsu G, et al. Radiographic distribution of *Pneumocystis carinii* pneumonia in patients with AIDS treated with prophylactic inhaled pentamidine. Radiology 1990; 175:715–19.

13. Sandhu JS, Goodman PC. Pulmonary cysts associated with *Pneumocystis carinii* pneumonia in patients with AIDS. Radiology 1989;173:33–5.

14. Kuhlman TE, Knowles MC, Fishman EK, Siegelman SS. Premature bullous pulmonary damage in AIDS: CT diagnosis. Radiology 1989;173:23–6.

15. Gurney JW, Bates FT. Pulmonary cystic disease: comparison of *Pneumocystis carinii* pneumatoceles and bullous emphysema due to intravenous drug abuse. Radiology 1989;173:27–31.

16. Schinella RA, Fazzini CC, et al. *Pneumocystis carinii* as a cause of pulmonary fibrosis. Am Rev Respir Dis 1986;133:180.

17. Sunderam G, Reichman LB. Tuberculosis and human immunodeficiency virus infection. Semin Respir Med 1988;9(5):481–5.

18. Pitchenik AE, Rubinson HA. The radiographic appearance of tuberculosis in patients with the acquired immunodeficiency syndrome. Am Rev Respir Dis 1985;131:393–6.

19. Glasroth J. *Mycobacterium avium* complex in patients with the acquired immunodeficiency syndrome. Semin Respir Med 1988;9(5):486–91.

20. O'Brian RJ. Pulmonary disease due to *mycobacterium avium* complex. Semin Respir Med 1988;9(5):492–7.

21. Jacobson MA. Mycobacterial diseases: tuberculosis and *mycobacterium avium* complex. Infect Dis Clin North Am 1988;2:465–74.

22. Young LS. *Mycobacterium avium* complex infection. J Infect Dis 1988;157:863–7.

23. Miller WS, Edelman JM, Miller WT. Cryptococcal pulmonary infection in patients with AIDS: radiographic appearance. Radiology 1990;175:725–8.

24. Balmes JR, Hawkins JG. Pulmonary cryptococcosis. Semin Respir Med 1987;9(2):180–6.

25. Gal AA, Koss MN, Hawkins J, et al. The pathology of pulmonary cryptococcal infections in the acquired immunodeficiency syndrome. Arch Pathol Lab Med 1986; 110:502–7.

26. Kuhlman JE, Fishman EK, Burch PAS, et al. CT of invasive pulmonary aspergillosis. AJR 1988;150:1015–20.

27. Chestnut TM, Ramsey PG. Pulmonary viral infections in the immunocompromised host. Semin Respir Med 1989;10(1):31–7.

28. Oliff JFC, Williams MP. Radiological appearances of cytomegalovirus infections. Clin Radiol 1989;40:463–7.

29. Graham BS, Snell JD. Herpes simplex virus infection of the adult lower respiratory tract. Medicine (Baltimore) 1983;62:384–494.

30. Ellison RF. Pulmonary bacterial infections in the immunocompromised host. Semin Respir Med 1989;10(1):38–47.

31. Amorosa JK, Nahass RG, Nosher JL, Gocke DJ. Radiologic distribution of pyogenic pulmonary infection from *Pneumocystis carinii* pneumonia in AIDS patients. Radiology 1990;175:721–4.

32. O'Brian RF. Pulmonary and pleural Kaposi's sarcoma in the acquired immunodeficiency syndrome. Semin Respir Med 1989;10(1):12–19.

33. Brown RKJ, Huberman RP, Vanley G. Pulmonary features of Kaposi's sarcoma. AJR 1982; 139:659–60.

34. Nyberg DA, Federle MP. AIDS-related Kaposi's sarcoma and lymphomas. Semin Roentgenol 1987;22(1):54–65.

35. Sivit CJ, Schwartz AM, Rockoff SD. Kaposi's sarcoma of the lung in AIDS: radiologic pathologic analysis. AJR 1987;148:25–8.

36. Zibrak JD, Silvestri RC, Costello P, et al. Bronchoscopic and radiologic features of Kaposi's sarcoma involving the respiratory system. Chest 1986;90(4):476–9.

37. Simmons JT, Suffredini AF, Lack EE, et al. Nonspecific interstitial pneumonitis in patients with AIDS: radiologic features. AJR 1987;149:265–8.

38. Suffredini AF, Ognibene FP, Lack EE, et al. Nonspecific interstitial pneumonitis; a common cause

of pulmonary disease in the acquired immuno-deficiency syndrome. Ann Intern Med 1987; 107: 7–13.

39. Grohman J, Kahn F. Noninfectious pulmonary disease in the immunocompromised host. Semin Respir Med 1989; 10(1): 78–88.

40. Corboy JR, Fink L, Miller WT. Congestive cardiomyopathy in association with AIDS. Radiology 1987; 165: 139–41.

41. Hover DE. Diagnosis of pulmonary disease in the immunocompromised host. Semin Respir Med 1989; 10(1): 100.

42. Miller RF, Millar AB, Weller IV, Semple SJ. Empirical treatment without bronchoscopy for *Pneumocystis carinii* pneumonia in the acquired immunodeficiency syndrome. Thorax 1989; 44: 559–64.

43. Auerbach DM, Harber P. Diagnostic approach to acquired immunodeficiency patients with pulmonary symptoms: a decision analytic strategy. Semin Respir Med 1989; 10(1): 252–7.

44. Mitchell DM. Diagnostic problems in AIDS and the lung. Respir Med 1989; 83: 9–14.

12 Endoscopic Examination of Gastrointestinal and Hepatobiliary Complications in Patients with HIV Infection

J. F. W. M. Bartelsman

Acute Primary HIV Infection

Primary infection with the human immunodeficiency virus type 1 (HIV-1) may be asymptomatic or associated with a flu-like or mononucleosis-like illness (1, 2). Gaines et al. describe the clinical picture of primary HIV infection in 20 consecutive patients, all male homosexuals (2). In the 10 patients for whom date of exposure to the virus could be established, the incubation period was 11–28 days (median 14). The mean duration of acute illness was 12.7 days. The clinical picture was characterized by a sudden onset of fever, sore throat, lymphadenopathy, rash, lethargy, dry cough, headache, myalgia, conjunctivitis, vomiting, nausea, and diarrhea. A particularly interesting finding in this study was the high incidence of painful, shallow ulcers in the mouth or on the genitals or anus. Five of the 20 patients had severe retrosternal pain when swallowing, but were not subjected to endoscopy.

In 12 patients from Sydney with acute HIV infection, esophageal symptoms were not mentioned (1). Only Kessler et al. describe endoscopic findings in one patient admitted with a 1-week history of fever and dysphagia (3); esophageal findings revealed four discrete ulcers whose biopsy showed inflammation and granulation tissue.

We diagnosed acute primary HIV esophagitis in a 29-year-old man who presented with fever, diarrhea, odynophagia, and a skin rash. Endoscopy of the esophagus revealed multiple small, shallow ulcerations resembling herpes simplex esophagitis, but herpes simplex virus could not be cultured from biopsy specimens. HIV-1-p24 antigen could only be shown in the blood on the first day of hospital admission, 7 days after the onset of the disease. Seroconversion for HIV-1 antibodies took place 28 days after the onset.

AIDS

A multitude of opportunistic infections and unusual malignancies has been documented in every organ system of patients with acquired immune deficiency syndrome.

About 50% of all AIDS patients have gastrointestinal manifestations with consequent morbidity and sometimes mortality (4). The gastrointestinal tract can be involved after infection with the human immunodeficiency virus in three different ways (5–8):

1. Opportunistic tumors: Kaposi's sarcoma, B-cell lymphoma, squamous carcinoma of the tongue and the anus
2. Opportunistic infections
3. Direct HIV effects on the gut

Over a 5-year period, 225 adult AIDS patients were seen at the Academic Medical Center (AMC) in Amsterdam. Three of the patients were female, 222 were male. The mean age was 38.3 years (21–63 years).

157 of these patients (70%) were found to have gastrointestinal disease by radiologic studies, endoscopy, laboratory tests, and by autopsy; 99 (44%) had diarrhea, 72 (32%) had dysphagia, primarily due to candidiasis, and 65 (29%) had Kaposi's sarcoma (KS) in the gastrointestinal tract. Anal pain due to herpes simplex infection (18%) was limited to homosexual men. In 42 (19%) of the patients, biliary or liver disease was diagnosed (Table 12.1).

Table 12.**1** Most frequent gastrointestinal abnormalities in 225 AIDS patients in the AMC

	n	%
Diarrhea	99	44
Dysphagia	72	32
Kaposi's sarcoma	65	29
Anal disease	40	18
Liver/biliary tract disease	42	19

Opportunistic (Viral) Tumors

Kaposi's sarcoma (KS) is frequently found in the gut of patients with cutaneous involvement (9). Postmortem studies show that the majority of patients with cutaneous KS have gut involvement and that lesions in the gastrointestinal tract may occur in the absence of any skin lesion (10).

KS can be in any part of the gastrointestinal tract and is mostly asymptomatic (11). Extensive involvement may lead to thickening of the intestinal wall, intestinal obstruction, and diarrhea.

The endoscopic picture of KS in the gut is:

1. small, flat, red or violet lesions (Fig. 12.**1**),
2. sessile red polyps, sometimes with a central ulceration (Figs. 12.**2**, 12.**3**),
3. larger tumors (Fig. 12.**4**).

Endoscopic biopsies frequently fail to make the diagnosis of KS, due to the submucosal nature of the majority of the KS lesions (5). Radiology mostly fails to show KS in the gut, because the lesions are often flat, but elevated lesions and thickening of the intestinal wall can be shown with barium examinations (12).

The therapeutic alternatives are:

1. Excision of localized lesions
2. Radiotherapy for the affected segment of the bowel
3. Chemotherapy
4. Interferon-α

Etoposide (VP-16) and vinblastine are used as "single agents." Combination chemotherapy effects a response in 30–80% of the patients, but remissions are incomplete and of short duration (13). Chemotherapy is often limited by concomitant opportunistic infections. Immunotherapy with interferon-α has considerable side-effects, such as fever and malaise (14). In our clinic, in patients with KS skin lesions, gastroduodenoscopy and rectosigmoidoscopy have been performed routinely before and during treatment with interferon-α.

In 65 of 225 AIDS patients at the AMC, we diagnosed one or more KS lesions in the gastrointestinal tract by endoscopy or autopsy (Table 12.**2**).

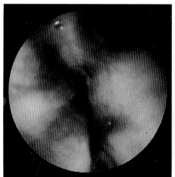 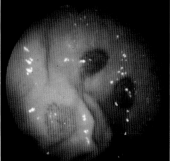 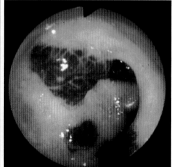

Fig. 12.**1**   Fig. 12.**2**   Fig. 12.**3**

Fig. 12.**1**   Flat KS lesions of the esophagus

Fig. 12.**2**   Multiple small polypoid KS lesions of the stomach

Fig. 12.**3**   Multiple elevated KS lesions of the stomach

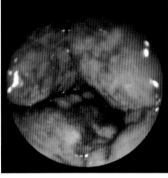
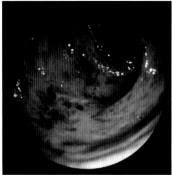
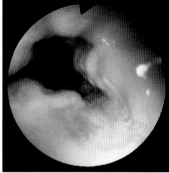

Fig. 12.**4**   Fig. 12.**5**   Fig. 12.**6**

Fig. 12.**4**   Large tumor mass due to KS of the rectum

Fig. 12.**5**   CMV colitis: multiple flat red lesions (intramucosal hemorrhage)

Fig. 12.**6**   CMV esophagitis

Table 12.**2**   KS lesions in the digestive tract of 65 patients in the AMC

Localization	Number of patients
Oropharynx	35
Esophagus	17
Stomach	36
Duodenum	21
Small intestine	13
Colon/rectum	26
Appendix	1

Non-Hodgkin's Lymphoma of the Bowel

NHLs, generally high-grade lymphomas of B cells, are often reported in homosexual AIDS patients (5, 15). NHL of the bowel can cause malabsorption, weight loss, diarrhea, and occasionally, perforation or bleeding (16). The prognosis of NHL in AIDS patients is very poor. In our hospital we saw three patients with NHL in the gastrointestinal tract (tonsil, stomach, and rectum).

Squamous Carcinoma

Squamous carcinoma of the tongue and cloacogenic carcinoma of the anus are described in homosexual AIDS patients, perhaps caused by a combination of local human papillomavirus (HPV) infection and systemic infection by HIV (5). Anal carcinoma was diagnosed in 2 of 225 AIDS patients in our clinic.

Gastrointestinal Infections

Viral Infections

Cytomegalovirus. CMV is a common cause of death in AIDS patients, particularly CMV infection of the lung and central nervous system. CMV can cause large, sharply demarcated ulcers in the esophagus and stomach or a diffuse gastritis (17). Ulcerations in the small intestine can lead to perforation (18).

The most important localization of CMV infection in the gastrointestinal tract is colitis. Patients with CMV colitis present with fever, watery diarrhea which is sometimes blood-streaked, abdominal distention, and abdominal pain. CMV may be isolated from the stools or from colonic biopsies. There are two different endoscopic pictures of CMV colitis:

1. multiple areas of red spots, caused by accumulations of erythrocytes in the mucosa (Fig. 12.**5**),
2. large ulcerations surrounded by normal mucosa (Figs. 12.**6**, 12.**7**).

Rectal or colonic biopsies can show the characteristic inclusion bodies of CMV.

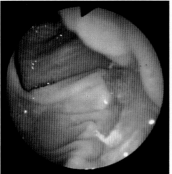 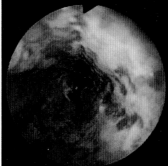 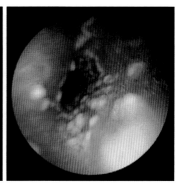

Fig. 12.**7**   Fig. 12.**8**   Fig. 12.**9**

Fig. 12.**7**   CMV colitis: large ulcer in the transverse colon

Fig. 12.**8**   Herpes esophagitis

Fig. 12.**9**   Moderate *Candida* esophagitis

In an evaluation of diagnostic criteria for mucosal CMV disease in AIDS patients, immunohistologic techniques proved to be more sensitive (92%) then viral cultures of the biopsies (only 30% positive; 19). IgG antibodies were not specific, and IgM antibodies were not sensitive and not specific.

The radiologic findings of CMV colitis are not specific and resemble ulcerative colitis (diffuse involvement) or Crohn's disease (segmental involvement; 20, 21).

Of 225 AIDS patients, 28 (12%) had complications of gastrointestinal CMV infection, mostly in the rectum or colon (Table 12.**3**).

Most patients with CMV complications respond to a treatment with dihydroxyproproxymethylguanine (DHPG; 17, 22). The drug works, similar to acyclovir, by decreasing viral replication. Usually long-term therapy is required.

Herpes simplex virus (Fig. 12.**8**). In homosexual male AIDS patients, it is common to find a past history of recurrent perianal herpes simplex infection. Perianal HSV ulcerations may be extremely extensive, involving large skin areas. Treatment with acyclovir (Zovirax) is highly effective, but long-term maintenance treatment is necessary to prevent recurrence (23; Table 12.**4**).

Table 12.**3**   CMV infections in the gastrointestinal tract of 28 patients in the AMC

Site	Number of patients
Esophagus	2
Stomach	5
Duodenum	6
Small intestine	2
Rectum/colon	12
Liver	5

Table 12.**4**   Viral infections in the digestive tract of 225 patients in the AMC

Infection	Number of patients	%
CMV	28	12
HSV (peri)anal	40	18
HSV esophagitis	2	0.9

Bacterial and Fungal Infections

Candidiasis. Oral candidiasis is frequently the earliest of the opportunistic infections and is a feature of AIDS-related complex (Figs. 12.**9**, 12.**10**). Esophageal candidiasis is caused by a greater degree of immunosuppression and is frequently seen in patients with AIDS. Symptoms of extension of *Candida* into the esophagus are dysphagia and weight loss.

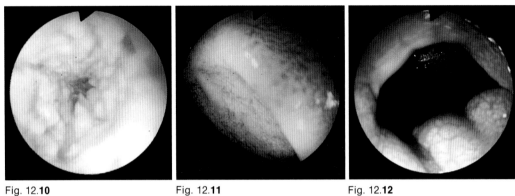

Fig. 12.**10**   Fig. 12.**11**   Fig. 12.**12**

Fig. 12.**10**   Severe *Candida* esophagitis

Fig. 12.**11**   MAI of the duodenum

Fig. 12.**12**   White thickened mucosa of the rectum due to MAI-containing macrophages

Table 12.**5**   Bacterial and fungal infections in the gastrointestinal tract of 225 AIDS patients in the AMC

Infection	Number of patients	%
Candida albicans	72	32
Salmonella typhimurium	8 ⎫ 9	4
Salmonella paratyphi	1 ⎭	
Shigella flexneri	3	1.3
Campylobacter jejuni	16	7.1
Yersinia enterocolitica	2	0.9
Mycobacterium avium – intercellulare	13	5.8
Mycobacterium tuberculosis	5	2.2

Oral candidiasis in ARC patients can be treated by topical antifungals, such as nystatin suspension or miconazole gel. In established AIDS and esophageal candidiasis, topical treatment alone is mostly insufficient and systemic antifungal treatment with ketoconazole or miconazole is required (24). Most patients need maintenance treatment to prevent recurrences.

In 225 AIDS patients in AMC we diagnosed esophageal candidiasis in about one-third of the patients (Table 12.**5**).

Bacterial infections. Persistent *Salmonella* infections, *Salmonella typhimurium* in parti-cular, are frequently described as a cause of diarrhea in AIDS patients (5).

Other pathogens, such as *Shigella flexneri*, *Campylobacter jejuni*, and *Yersinia entero-colitica* are also often clutured from the stools of AIDS patients (Table 12.**5**).

Infection with *Mycobacterium tuberculosis* is considered a reactivation of latent infection. Bowel infection with *Mycobacterium tuberculosis* may present a typical pattern of ileocaecal involvement and commonly leads to enlargement of mesenteric lymph nodes. Infection with *Mycobacterium avium–intracellulare* (MAI) is seen in a later stage of AIDS, and may occur in any part of the bowel and lead to severe diarrhea, malabsorption, and weight loss (Figs. 12.**11**, 12.**12**).

The histologic picture of MAI enteritis can resemble Whipple's disease, characterized by PAS-positive macrophages containing acid-fast bacteria (25, 26). Infections with MAI respond poorly to common antituberculous drugs.

Protozoal Infection

Infections with *Giardia lamblia* are frequently diagnosed in patients with AIDS and can easily be treated with metronidazole. More specific AIDS-related infections are caused

Table 12.**6** Protozoal infections in the gastro-intestinal tract of 225 AIDS patients in the AMC

Infection	Number of patients	%
Entamoeba histolytica	17	7.5
Giardia lamblia	19	8.4
Cryptosporidium	17	7.5
Isospora belli	1	0.4

Table 12.**7** Causes of elevated liver enzyme levels in the blood and/or jaundice in 225 AIDS patients in the AMC

CMV hepatitis	5
Mycobacterium avium – intracellulare	6
Mycobacterium tuberculosis	1
Chronic active hepatitis B	7
Acute hepatitis B	1
Liver cirrhosis	1
Chronic non-A, non-B hepatitis	1
Hepatotoxic drug	5
Kaposi's sarcoma	5

by *Cryptosporidium* and *Isospora belli*, two protozoal parasites of the Coccidia order (Table 12.**6**). Both parasites cause severe diarrhea, malabsorption, and weight loss and are not amenable to therapy (27, 28).

Cryptosporidium infects the small bowel. The parasite lies in the microvilli of the epithelium and leads to villous atrophy. *Isospora belli* lies within the columnar cells.

The diagnosis of both Coccidia infections can be made by showing the parasites in duodenal or jejunal biopsies, or by the finding of oocysts in fresh stool specimens.

Liver and Biliary Disease

Patients with AIDS commonly have clinical and histologic hepatic abnormalities (31; Table 12.7):

1. concomitant hepatitis B,
2. opportunistic infections,
3. opportunistic tumors,
4. iatrogenic complications,
5. nonspecific changes associated with chronic illness.

Hepatitis B Virus and AIDS

Markers of past hepatitis B infection are found in approximately 90% of AIDS patients. The prevalence of chronic HBV infection is about 10% (31). Chronic active hepatitis and cirrhosis appear to be unusual, probably because liver cell damage in HBV infections is dependent on the host's cellular immunity.

Hepatic Infections

The most commonly diagnosed hepatic infection in AIDS is caused by *Mycobacterium avium – intracellulare*, which can be found in granulomas, in histiocytes, or in Kupffer cells. Hepatic granulomas can also be found secondary to *Mycobacterium* tuberculosis or histoplasmosis, sometimes also to toxoplasmosis or CMV hepatitis. Acute hepatitis can be caused by the CMV, herpes simplex virus, or Epstein–Barr virus (31–34).

Infections of the biliary tract with CMV or *Cryptosporidium* may result in acalculous cholecystitis or focal strictures in the bile ducts, resembling primary sclerosing cholangitis (35).

Opportunistic Tumors

When the liver is involved in KS, the tumor is generally widely disseminated in multiple organs (31). The liver may be involved by malignant lymphoma of a monoclonal B-cell type.

Iatrogenic Complications

AIDS patients are exposed to numerous potential hepatotoxic drugs. Of 225 AIDS patients in the AMC, 42 had elevated blood levels of alkaline phosphatase and transaminase during their illness, 9 also had jaundice.

In many cases, a specific diagnosis was not made because no liver biopsy had been performed. Liver biopsy had not been attempted because of the bad general condition of the patient or because the elevated liver enzyme levels were only transient. The well-documented liver and biliary tract abnormalities are summarized in Table 12.7. The hepatotoxic drugs were Daraprim (pyrimethamine), isoniazid (INH), pentamidine, Nizoral (ketoconazole), and Diphantoine (phenytoin).

Conclusions

Patients with acute primary HIV infection can complain of retrosternal pain on swallowing. Painful ulcers in the mouth, on the genitals or anus and in the esophagus have been described. Gastrointestinal complications are found in the majority of patients with AIDS. Main gastrointestinal symptoms are dysphagia, abdominal pain, diarrhea, and signs of perianal disease. Dysphagia is mostly caused by esophageal candidiasis; perianal disease is mainly due to HSV.

Diarrhea and malabsorption can be caused by many viral, bacterial, or protozoal infections that can be diagnosed by examination of stool specimens or by cultures and histologic examination of duodenal and colonic biopsies. Some intestinal infections require long-term treatment. Unfortunately other infections (MAI, *Cryptosporidium*, *Isospora belli*) are not amenable to specific therapy and can only be treated by supportive measures.

In our hospital, 359 gastrointestinal endoscopies were performed in 137 of 225 AIDS patients (60%): 193 gastroduodenoscopies and 166 sigmoidoscopies or colonoscopies.

References

1. Cooper DA, Gold J, Maclean P, et al. Acute AIDS retrovirus infection: definition of clinical illness associated with seroconversion. Lancet 1985; i: 537–40.
2. Gaines H, von Sydow M, Pehrson PO, Lundbergh P. Clinical picture of primary HIV infection presenting as a glandular fever–like illness. BMJ 1988; 297: 1363–8.
3. Kessler HA, Blaauw B, Spaar J, Paul DA, Falk LA, Landay A. Diagnosis of human immunodeficiency virus infection in seronegative homosexuals presenting with an acute viral syndrome. JAMA 1987; 258: 1196–9.
4. Santangelo WC, Krejs GJ. Southwestern internal medicine conference: gastrointestinal manifestations of the acquired immunodeficiency syndrome. Am J Med Sci 1986; 292: 328–34.
5. Weber J. Gastrointestinal disease in AIDS: clinics in immunology and allergy 1986; 3: 519–41.
6. Gelb A, Miller S. Clinical reviews: AIDS and gastroenterology. Am J Gastroenterol 1986; 81: 619–22.
7. Gillin JS, Shike M, Alcock N, et al. Malabsorption and mucosal abnormalities of the small intestine in the acquired immunodeficiency syndrome. Ann Intern Med 1985; 102: 619–22.
8. Smith PD, Lane HC, Gill VJ, Manischewitz JF, Quinnan GV, Fanci AS, Masur H. Intestinal infections in patients with the acquired immunodeficiency syndrome (AIDS). Ann Intern Med 1988; 108: 328–33.
9. Saltz RK, Kurtz RC, Lightdale CJ, et al. Kaposi's sarcoma: gastrointestinal involvement, correlation with skin findings and immunological function. Dig Dis Sci 1984; 29: 817–23.
10. Lemlich G, Schwam L, Lebwohl M. Kaposi's sarcoma and acquired immunodeficiency syndrome: postmortem findings in twenty-four cases. J Am Acad Dermatol 1987; 16: 319–25.
11. Ell C, Matek W, Gramatzki M, Kaduk B, Demling L. Endoscopic findings in a case of Kaposi's sarcoma with involvement of the large and small bowel. Endoscopy 1985; 17: 161–4.
12. Wall SD, Friedman SL, Margulis AR. Gastrointestinal Kaposi's sarcoma in AIDS: radiographic manifestations. J Clin Gastroenterol 1984; 6: 165–71.
13. Smith N, Spittle M. ABC of AIDS tumours. Br Med J 1987; 1274–7.
14. Krown SE, Real FX, Cunningham-Rundles S, Myskowski PL, Koziner B, Fein S, Mittelman A, Oeltgen HF, Safai B. Preliminary observations on the effect of recombinant leukocyte A interferon in homosexual men with Kaposi's sarcoma. N Engl J Med 1983; 308: 1071–6.
15. Levine AM, Gill PS, Meyer PR. Retrovirus and malignant lymphoma in homosexual men. JAMA 1985; 254: 1921–5.
16. Robinson G, Wilson SE, Williams RA. Surgery in patients with acquired immunodeficiency syndrome. Arch Surg 1987; 122: 170–5.
17. Dieterich DT. Cytomegalovirus: a new gastrointestinal pathogen in immunocompromised patients (editorial). Am J Gastroenterol 1987; 82: 764–5.
18. Houin HP, Gruenberg JC, Fisher EJ, Mezger E. Multiple small bowel perforations secondary to cytomegalovirus in a patient with acquired im-

munodeficiency syndrome. Henry Ford Hosp Med J 1987; 35:17–19.

19. Culpepper-Morgan JA, Kotler DP, Scholes JV, Tierney AR. Evaluation of diagnostic criteria for mucosal cytomegalic inclusion disease in the acquired immune deficiency syndrome. Am J Gastroenterol 1987; 82:1264–70.

20. Balthazar EJ, Magibow AJ, Fazzini E, Opulencia JF, Engel I. Cytomegalovirus colitis in AIDS: radiographic findings in 11 patients. Radiology 1985; 155:585–9.

21. Frager DH, Frager JD, Wolf EL, et al. Cytomegalovirus colitis in acquired immune deficiency syndrome: radiologic spectrum. Gastrointest Radiol 1986; 11:241–6.

22. Bach MC, Bapwell SP, Knapp NP. DHPG for CMV infections in patients with AIDS. Ann Intern Med 1985; 103:381–2.

23. Straus SE, Seidlin M, Takiff H. Oral acyclovir to suppress recurring herpes simplex virus infection in immunodeficient patients. Ann Intern Med 1984; 100:522–4.

24. Deschamps MMH, Pape JW, Verdier RI, DeHovitz J, Thomas F, Johnson WD. Treatment of *Candida* esophagitis in AIDS patients. Am J Gastroenterol 1988; 83:20–1.

25. Roth RI, Owen RL, Keren DF, Volberding PA. Intestinal infection with *Mycobacterium avium* in acquired immune deficiency syndrome (AIDS): histological and clinical comparison with Whipple's disease. Dig Dis Sci 1985; 30:497–504.

26. Kooijman CD, Poen H. Whipple-like disease in AIDS (correspondence). Histopathology 1984; 8:705–7.

27. Modigliani R, Bories C, Le Charpentier Y, et al. Diarrhoea and malabsorption in acquired immune deficiency syndrome, a study of four cases with special emphasis on opportunistic protozoan infestations. Gut 1985; 26:179–87.

28. Berg RN, Wall SD, McArdle CB, et al. Cryptosporidiosis of the stomach and small intestine in patients with AIDS. Am J Radiology 1984; 143:549–54.

29. Shein R, Gelb A. *Isospora belli* in a patient with acquired immunodeficiency syndrome. J Clin Gastroenterol 1984; 6:525–8.

30. Forthal DN, Guest SS. *Isospora belli* enteritis in three homosexual men. Am J Trop Med Hyg 1984; 33:1060–4.

31. Lebovics E, Dworkin BM, Heier SK, Rosenthal WS. The hepatobiliary manifestations of human immunodeficiency virus infection. Am J Gastroenterol 1988; 83:1–7.

32. Dworkin BM, Stahl RE, Giardina MA, Wormser GP, Weiss L, Jankowski R, Rosenthal WS. The liver in acquired immune deficiency syndrome: emphasis on patients with intravenous drug abuse. Am J Gastroenterol 1987; 82:231–6.

33. Kahn SA, Saltzman BR, Klein RS, Mahadevia PS, Friedland GH, Brandt LJ. Hepatic disorders in the acquired immune deficiency syndrome: a clinical and pathological study. Am J Gastroenterol 1986; 81:1145–8.

34. Glasgow BJ, Anders K, Layfield LJ, Steinsapir KD, Gitnick GL, Lewin KJ. Clinical and pathological findings of the liver in the acquired immune deficiency syndrome (AIDS). Am J Clin Pathol 1985; 83:582–8.

35. Margulis SJ, Honig CL, Soave R, Govoni AF, Mouzadian JA, Jacobson IM. Biliary tract obstruction in the acquired immunodeficiency syndrome. Ann Intern Med 1986; 105:207–10.

13 Radiology of Gastrointestinal Manifestations in AIDS

J. W. A. J. Reeders, A. J. Megibow, H. R. Antonides

GI disease accounts for the second largest overall group of diseases (after *Pneumocystis carinii* pneumonia) seen in AIDS patients (1–7). Candidiasis, cytomegalovirus (CMV), cryptosporidiosis, histoplasmosis, isosporiasis, salmonella (with sepsis), and unusual mycobacteria account for a majority of nonneoplastic disorders (8). Neoplasms include Kaposi's sarcoma (KS), and high-grade non-Hodgkin's B-cell lymphomas (NHL). Multiple sites may be involved in significant numbers of patients (9). Several entities display radiographic features allowing for a specific diagnosis. The predominant radiographic pattern may indicate which particular entity is most accountable for clinical symptomatology at the time of examination. As radiologic experience accumulates, these patterns will become more clearly defined (10, 11).

Radiographic Technique

Wall et al. (11) have shown that double-contrast studies more frequently detected abnormalities (95% of the 40 patients examined) when compared to single-contrast studies, which detected abnormalities in 61% of 23 patients examined. We recommend the routine use of double-contrast radiographic techniques in the study of the esophagus, stomach, and colon. Many excellent texts and articles review the methodology by which these studies may be performed (11–19).

Abdominal CT scans should be performed using sufficient oral contrast material to ensure uniform bowel opacification. Air-contrast methodology aids in the detection of gastric, esophagogastric, and colonic lesions. At least 800 mL, consumed evenly over a 30- to 45-minute period before the scan begins, will generally provide uniform bowel opacification.

Intravenous (IV) contrast enhancement should be utilized in all cases (unless contraindicated by allergy or renal disease). Contrast is administered in two phases: a rapid bolus (50 mL) is followed immediately by sustained infusion of the remaining contrast (100–150 mL), which is maintained as the scans are acquired. Scans are obtained using a dynamic sequential protocol that maximizes intravascular contrast levels. This increases the accuracy of detection of intrahepatic masses and discrimination of lymph nodes from vessels in the retroperitoneum and mesentery (20).

Esophagus

Nonneoplastic Lesions

Esophagitis

Dysphagia is a common complaint in AIDS patients. Monilial, CMV, and herpes infections account for the significant percentage of cases. Radiographic assessment is useful for several reasons:

1. *Candida* and CMV infections can be differentiated radiographically
2. The radiographic pattern may suggest a diagnosis necessitating aggressive endoscopic biopsy and culture techniques
3. Therapeutic response can be assessed objectively

Candidiasis is the most common cause of esophagitis in AIDS patients (2). Oral thrush may be seen in patients with AIDS-related complex (ARC), but diffuse esophageal *Candida* infection is a manifestation of "full-blown" AIDS (21; Figs. 13.**1**, 13.**2**). According to the Centers for Disease Control (CDC) case surveillance criteria, candidiasis of the

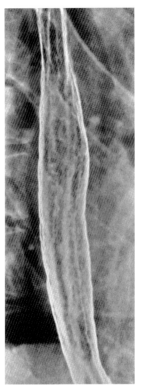
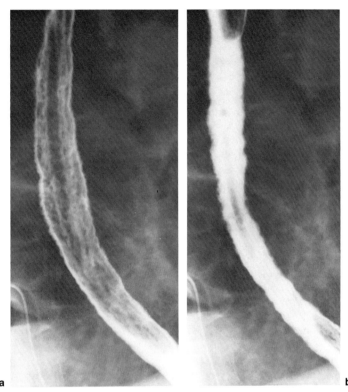

a

b

Fig. 13.**1**   Mild *Candida* esophagitis

Fig. 13.**2**   Severe *Candida* esophagitis "shaggy esophagus". **a** Double contrast (DC), **b** Single contrast (SC) esophagogram

esophagus may be considered presumptive evidence for the diagnosis of AIDS in patients with laboratory evidence of HIV infection. Frager found candidiasis to be the most common AIDS-related GI infection (12/25 patients; 2). Similarly, Wall et al. encountered *Candida* infection in 15 of 44 patients (11).

Radiographic appearances vary according to the severity of the disease (13–16; Table 13.1). Classically, candidiasis results in a diffusely ulcerated shaggy esophagus (22, 23). Other forms include cobblestoning, plaques, and thickened mucosal folds (17, 24). Levine et al. (17) showed the double-contrast esophagography is more sensitive in detecting esophageal candidiasis than single-contrast esophagography, with accuracy of detection approaching 90%. This improved accuracy reflects the ability to detect mucosal plaques that may be focally clustered, pro-

ducing longitudinally oriented linear filling defects (16, 18). This pattern accounted for 95% of the *Candida* lesions seen on double-contrast studies (17).

CMV Esophagitis

CMV esophagitis displays several unique appearances. CMV, a variety of herpesvirus, can be transmitted in humans by contaminated urine, secretions, blood transfusion, and sexual contact. Frequently involved organs include lungs, adrenals, liver, and spleen. The GI tract, pancreas, and biliary tree are affected more rarely (3, 25–31). The colon seems to be the organ most commonly affected; involvement of stomach and small intestine is less frequent (3, 25–27, 32). Focal, discretely marginated diamond-shaped ulcers surrounded by a well-defined peripheral lu-

Table 13.1   Spectrum of radiologic features in AIDS of the esophagus

Organism/disease	Radiologic features	Extent of disease
Nonneoplastic lesions		
	Mild	Generally diffuse;
Candidiasis	Edematous mucosal folds	sometimes focal
	Minimal plaques	
	Ulceration	
	Moderate	
	Edematous mucosal folds	
	Diffuse plaque formation	
	Fine ulceration	
	Severe	
	Thickened mucosal folds	
	Diffuse deep longitudinal ulcerations	
	Extensive diffuse or focally clustered plaques ("shaggy esophagus")	
	Cobblestoning	
	Pseudomembranes	
	End stage	
	Polypoid lesions	
	Mucosal "bridging"	
	Strictures	
CMV	Shallow, poorly defined or focally discretely marginated diamond shaped ulcers with well-defined peripheral lucency (edema) on normal mucosal background	Focal or diffuse
	Irregular thickening of mucosal folds	Predilection for esophago-gastric junction
	Giant esophageal longitudinally shaped ulcers	
	CT Thickening of abdominal part of esophagus	
	Increased density of lesser omental fat	
HSV	Similar to CMV	Focal or diffuse
Mycobacterium		
Mycobacterium avium – intracellulare (MAI)	Longitudinal ulceration	Focal
Mycobacterium tuberculosis	Sinus tracts to mediastinum	

Table 13.**1**   (Continued)

Organism/disease	Radiologic features	Extent of disease
Neoplasms		
Kaposi's sarcoma	Thickening of mucosal folds	Diffuse
	Discrete sharp submucosal nodules (5 mm − 2 cm) with or without central umbilication	
	Normal intervening mucosa	
	No ulceration	
	CT Multiple filling defects	
	Obliteration of parapharyngeal spaces	

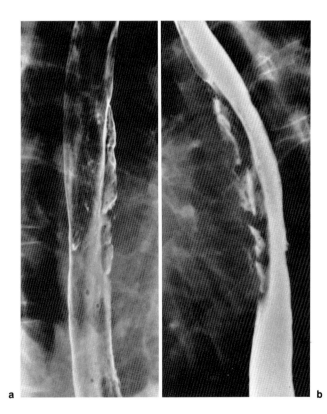

Fig. 13.**3**   CMV esophagitis. Longitudinal semilunar deep penetrated ulceration at the midesophagus. **a** DC, **b** SC esophagogram (tangential view)

cency representing zones of edema against a background of normal esophageal mucosa is seen (Fig. 13.3). Balthazar et al. (13) described discrete lesions along the length of the esophagus in 16 cases of CMV esophagitis. Teixidor et al. (33) reported four cases of CMV esophagitis, and in three cases the diagnoses were missed on single-contrast studies.

There is a high incidence of ulcerations at the gastroesophageal junction with extension of the process into the proximal stomach.

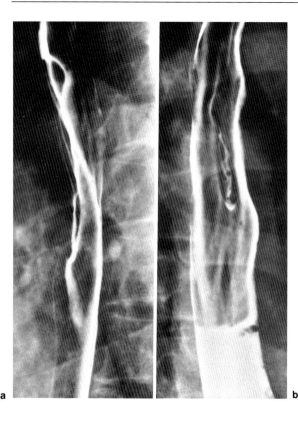

a

b

Fig. 13.**4** *Mycobacterium* esophagitis. Longitudinal deep ulceration at the proximal esophagus. **a** tangential view, **b** AP view

This may be seen on CT scans as thickening of the abdominal portion of the esophagus and increased density in the lesser omental fat.

Giant esophageal ulcers may occur. This phenomenon results from a combination of infectious destruction of the mucosa and ischemic necrosis induced by vasculitis resulting from CMV infection of the endothelial cells in the submucosal blood vessels (34).

Farman et al. (14) recently described focal *Candida* lesions in 4 of 25 patients resulting in large esophageal ulcers. In our experience it is unusual to see large focal ulcers surrounded by normal mucosa in candidiasis. Contrast examination of the esophagus is characteristic of CMV infection.

Herpes Esophagitis

Herpes simplex esophagitis (HSV type 1) accounts for the second major etiology of esophageal infection in AIDS patients. The findings of discrete ulceration are similar to those seen with CMV in contrast to the diffuse ulcerations seen in *Candida* (15, 18, 35–37). In advanced stages the lesions may be indistinguishable from CMV. We have seen aggressive bacterial esophagitides in these patients as well.

Mycobacterium Esophagitis

Mycobacterial infections of the GI tract are being seen with increasing frequency due in large part to the AIDS epidemic. Both *M. tuberculosis* and atypical mycobacterial infections may be encountered (38).

MAI is a ubiquitous environmental contaminant rarely producing disease even in patients immunosuppressed due to other causes. This infection has been seen in 20% of AIDS patients followed by the National Institutes of Health (39). Haitians with AIDS showed a 60% prevalence of tuberculosis (*M. tuberculosis* and *M. avium–intracellulare*) versus a 2.7% prevalence in non-Haitian AIDS patients (40, 41). The organism is disseminated in the lung, liver, spleen, bone marrow, lymph nodes, and GI tract. MAI has a high morbidity and mortality rate (30, 42, 43). Mycobacterial esophagitis is a rare disease, usually occurring in the late stages of pulmonary tuberculosis (44) (Fig. 13.**4**).

Histologic examination of the intestine reveals large, "foamy" histiocytes in the lamina propria. Acid-fast staining demonstrates the cells to be filled with numerous bacilli. Lack of granuloma formation is characteristic of AIDS-related MAI infection (45).

Neoplasms

Kaposi's Sarcoma

The original observation of KS goes back to 1872, when Moritz Kaposi described it as a rare form of multiple hemorrhagic skin lesions (46). It is characterized by the "appearance of multiple small macules, blue or purplish, that slowly coalesce to form larger lesions."

Patients with AIDS and AIDS-related disorders are predisposed to developing KS (43, 47, 48).

In a clinicopathologic study of 56 autopsies by Niedt et al., 52% of patients with AIDS had KS (49). For unknown reasons the incidence of KS is much higher among homosexual men (44%) than in other AIDS patients (intravenous drug abusers, 4%; 4, 5, 43). Visible cutaneous or oral lesions are seen in 95% of AIDS patients with KS (50, 51). Common sites of involvement included skin (93%), lymph nodes (72%), lungs (52%), liver (34%), and rarely, the brain. The GI tract was involved in 48% (49, 52).

KS accounts for the majority of AIDS-related neoplasms in the esophagus and hypopharynx (53, 54). KS lesions are discrete, submucosal elevations seen along the length of the esophagus (Fig. 13.**5**). Hypo-

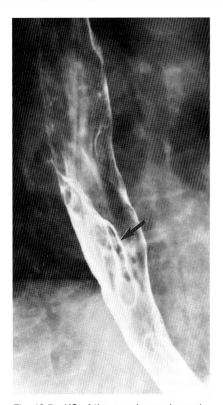

Fig. 13.**5**   KS of the esophagus (arrow)

pharyngeal KS lesions are significant sources of dysphagia due to their location and may be encountered in patients being studied to rule out esophagitis (52). The lesions may appear as small nodules or infiltrating masses. In CT scanning, multiple filling defects distorting the structures of the hypopharynx can be recognized. Obliteration of parapharyngeal spaces may be appreciated in infiltrating forms of the disease.

Stomach

Most gastric lesions are serendipitiously detected. The radiologist may be the first to detect gastric diseases in AIDS patients (Table 13.**2**). In the series by Wall et al. (11), gastric lesions were detected in 57% of patients; in that by Frager et al. (2), gastric pathology was found in 2 of 25 patients.

Table 13.**2** Spectrum of radiologic features in AIDS of the stomach

Organism/disease	Radiologic features	Extent of disease
Nonneoplastic lesions		
CMV	Irregular thickening of mucosal folds	Focal or diffuse
	Lack of distensibility	Predilection for the antrum
	Tiny ulcerations and granularity of mucosa	
	Narrowing of lumen	
Mycobacterium	Ulcerations	Segmental
Mycobacterium avium – intracellulare (MAI)	Hypertrophic fibrotic encasement	Predilection for the antrum
Mycobacterium tuberculosis	Gastric bulky mass extending into the mesenterium	
Cryptosporidium	Lack of distensibility	Segmental
	Rigidity	
	Deformity	Predilection for the antrum
	Thickening of mucosal folds	
Neoplasms		
Kaposi's sarcoma	Thickening of mucosal folds	Focal or diffuse
	Discrete, sharply defined submucosal nodules (5 mm – 2 cm) with or without central umbilication	
	"Thumbprinting"	
	Normal intervening mucosa	
	Overlying mucosa: ulcerated	
	Narrowing of the lumen	
	CT Thickening of the gastric wall with peripheral lucency (submucosal edema)	
Non-Hodgkin's lymphoma	Polypoid lesions, simulating adenocarcinoma	Focal
	Loss of mucosal pattern	Predisposition for the antrum
	Blunting of mucosal folds	
	Deep, well-defined penetrating ulcers	
	Narrowing of the lumen	
	CT Variable thickening of stomach wall/folds	
	Loss of mucosa	
	Mesenteric lymphadenopathy: infrequent	

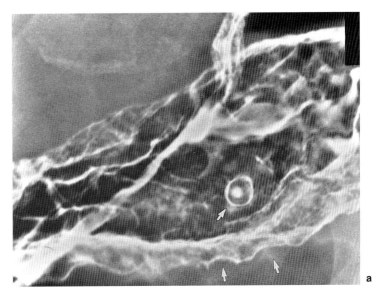

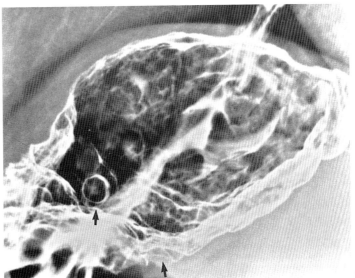

Fig. 13.**6**   KS of the stomach. Thickening of mucosal folds; submucosal nodules with (arrow) and without umbilication

Nonneoplastic Lesions

Nonneoplastic lesions are seen most often at the gastroesophageal junction and juxtapyloric antrum. Patients with CMV gastritis are referred to exclude malignancy (25, 27, 55). Many patients are examined by CT in search of signs of malignant disease. The radiologist must scrutinize the gastroesophageal junction region and antrum for signs of wall thickening. The CT findings are nonspecific; wall thickening should signal the need for barium radiography and/or endoscopy.

The antrum is the most frequent site of involvement. Submucosal lesions may produce "thumbprinting" along the gastric wall. This may be distinguished from the less regular, more discrete submucosal masses in

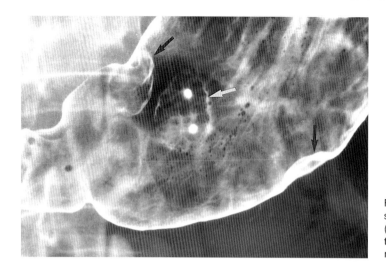

Fig. 13.**7** KS of the stomach: sharp submucosal nodules (arrows) with central umbilication on normal intervening mucosa

KS. In CT, the gastric wall is thickened, with a lucent appearance reflecting submucosal edema.

Gastric tuberculosis (*Mycobacterium tuberculosis*) with lesser omental abscess (56) has been reported. It occurs less often than enterocolic tuberculosis (38, 57).

Monilial bezoars have been demonstrated in patients with severe *Candida* infections of both the stomach and esophagus.

Neoplasms

Kaposi's Sarcoma

KS is commonly seen in the stomach of AIDS patients (58). Most but not all patients (93%) have skin lesions. Gastric lesions are best detected in double-contrast studies (59). CT scanning is not indicated in detecting gastric KS, although the lesions may be seen on carefully performed studies.

The radiographic finding is one or more discrete, sharply margined, submucosal nodules that are variable in size, but generally measure between 0.5 and 2 cm (Figs. 13.**6**, 13.**7**). The mucosa overlying the nodule may be ulcerated. Serial examinations may document progressive infiltration of the submucosa (Fig. 13.**8**).

Non-Hodgkin's Lymphoma

NHLs, generally high-grade lymphomas of B-cells with a poor prognosis, occur approximately one-tenth as often as KS (60). However, present figures may underestimate the future incidence of NHLs based on the estimated several million individuals who have already been infected with the AIDS virus (5, 6).

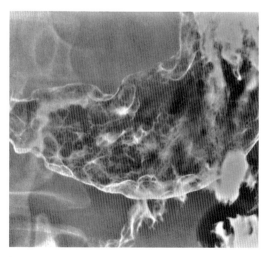

Fig. 13.**8a** KS of corpus and antrum of the stomach; multiple submucosal nodules are visible after barium meal

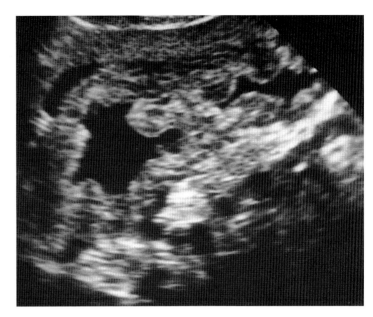

Fig. 13.**8b** Ultrasonography
stomach: disseminated
Kaposi's sarcoma in AIDS;
note the transmural infiltration
of the stomach wall by KS.
Courtesy: S. R. Wilson, M.D.,
FRCP(C) The Toronto Hospital,
Toronto, Canada

The GI tract is a common site of involvement for AIDS-related lymphoma (22–33%; 61–64). Although any portion of the GI tract may be involved, oral, rectal, and distal ileal sites are most frequently affected. Involvement of the stomach is rare (Fig. 13.**9**).

Duodenum and Small Bowel

Duodenal and small-intestinal disease accounts for the greatest percentage of GI abnormalities seen radiographically in AIDS patients. Wall et al. (11) found duodenal abnormality in 82%, jejunal abnormality in 64%, and ileal disease in 46% of 28 AIDS patients with upper GI abnormalities. Frager et al. (2) reported small-bowel disease in 13 of 25 patients. Organisms commonly causing enteritis include CMV and *Mycobacterium avium–intracellulare* and *Cryptosporidium*. KS and lymphoma are commonly seen neoplasms.

The clinical setting in which the small bowel will be examined includes those patients with diarrhea or malabsorption, or those patients in whom severe and rapid weight loss, pain, and fever suggests neoplas-

tic involvement. In a prospective evaluation of 22 AIDS patients with diarrhea and/or malabsorption, 10 had infections (Cryptosporidia, 3; MAI, 3; campylobacter, 2; candidiasis, 1; salmonella, 1). In two of five patients with malabsorption, no organism was found despite the presence of striking villous atrophy (56).

Radiologic evaluation is based on the distribution of disease, the presence or absence of distorsion of the small-bowel folds, the presence or absence of nodularity, and changes in the small-bowel caliber (Table 13.**3**).

Nonneoplastic Lesions

Cryptosporidiosis

Cryptosporidium—a small parasitic protozoon of 2–6μm—has shown to be an important cause of severe infections of the small bowel in patients with disordered immunoregulation associated with AIDS.

Cryptosporidial infections may produce a variable pattern of clinical symptoms ranging from moderately severe diarrhea to a cholera-like illness that results in uncontrollable de-

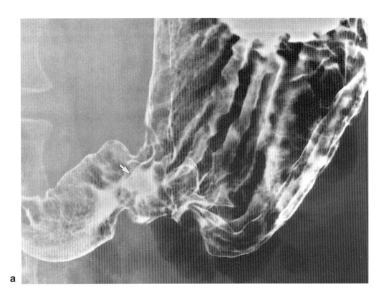

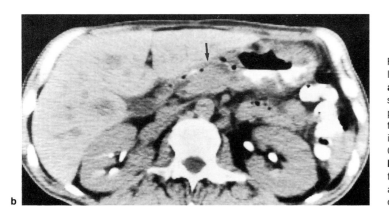

Fig. 13.**9** Non-Hodgkin's lymphoma of the stomach.
a Double-contrast barium study of the stomach: nodular protrusions into the lumen of the proximal antrum, simulating adenocarcinoma. Deep CMV ulcer (arrow)
b CT: Polypoid lesions protruding into the lumen of the antrum, simulating adenocarcinoma (arrow)

hydration, fluid and electrolyte disturbances, and even death (31, 65–68). Diagnosis is based on identification of the acid-fast staining oocysts in the stool. Endoscopic biopsy reveals organisms along the brush border of the intestinal microvilli. Treatment has had limited success, although spiramycin (an anti-toxoplasma antibiotic) has provided some control (59). Recently, bovine transfer factors have been used with varying results. Cases of dissemination to the lungs, spleen, and biliary tree have been reported (66).

Berk et al. reported on barium studies in 16 patients, 13 of which were abnormal: five patients showed thickened folds in the proximal small bowel, four showed fragmentation, three had spasm, and one showed mild dilatation. Most of the involvement was in the proximal intestine with marked thickening and hypersecretion present in the duodenum and jejunum (Fig. 13.**10**). In two cases gastric involvement was also present (65). Of note is the high predilection for associated thickening of folds in the duodenum. Differential diagnosis include giardiasis, strongyloidosis, Zollinger–Ellison syndrome, cystic fibrosis, acquired hypogammaglobulinemia, and alpha chain disease. *Isospora*

Table 13.**3**   Spectrum of radiologic features in AIDS of the duodenum/small bowel

Organism/disease	Radiologic features	Extent of disease
Nonneoplastic lesions		
Cryptosporidium	Spasm, irritability	Segmental
	Marked dilatation	
	Thickening of mucosal folds	Predilection for the
	Mucosal villous atrophy	duodenum/jejunum
	Marked nodularity	
	Marked hypersecretion	
	Fragmentation of barium	
Mycobacterium		
Mycobacterium avium –	Mild dilatation	Segmental
intracellulare (MAI)	Uniform thickening of valvulae	
Mycobacterium tuberculosis	conniventes	Predilection for the proximal
	Spasm, irregularity	jejunum
	Fine nodularity	
	Mild hypersecretion	
	Fragmentation of barium	
	"Pseudo Whipple"	
CMV	Mild dilatation	Focal or diffuse
	Thickening of valvulae	
	conniventes	Predilection for the terminal ileum
	Submucosal nodules	
	(0.25–0.75 cm)	
	Separation of loops	
	Discrete to deep round or	
	serpiginous ulcerations of	
	various size/depth	
	Fistula	
	Narrowing of the lumen	
	Obstruction	
	Perforation	
	CT Thickening of the intestinal	
	wall associated with colonic	
	disease	

belli, another coccidial protozoon, may produce identical radiologic features.

Mycobacterium

In the small bowel, MAI infection may produce a "pseudo-Whipple" appearance (69–72).

Vincent and Robbins (73) describe the radiographic findings that consisted of mild dilatation of the small bowel with thick undulating folds and fine nodularity. CT scanning reveals mesenteric and retroperitoneal lymphadenopathy, splenomegaly, and ascites (42). The nodes may demonstrate low-density regions in approximately 33% of cases.

Cytomegalovirus

CMV infection of the small bowel results in a diffuse enteritis or ileocolitis (11, 12). It is a

Table 13.**3**   (Continued)

Organism/disease	Radiologic features	Extent of disease
Neoplasms		
Kaposi's sarcoma	Thickening of mucosal folds	Diffuse
	Discrete sharp submucosal nodules (1–2 cm)	
	Normal intervening mucosa	
	Narrowing of the lumen	
Non-Hodgkin's lymphoma	Polypoid lesions, simulating adenocarcinoma	Focal
	Loss of mucosal pattern	Predisposition for the area distal to the ligament of Treitz and for the distal ileum
	Thickening/blunting of folds between polypoid lesions	
	Discrete, deep penetrating ulcers	
	Narrowing of the lumen	
	CT Variable thickening of small-bowel loops	
	Loss of mucosal pattern	
	Blunting of folds	
	Mesenteric lymphadenopathy: infrequent	

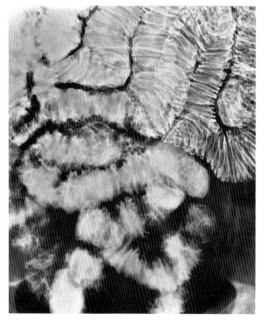

Fig. 13.**10** *Cryptosporidium* infection of the small bowel; thickening of mucosal folds

severe manifestation of AIDS and it may be preterminal. Intestinal perforation may occur (70) and is attributed to the ischemic necrosis secondary to vasculitis induced by CMV inclusion bodies found in the endothelial cells and the small vessels in the bowel wall (32).

In barium radiography, CMV may produce a diffuse enteritis, but in our experience it more commonly produces findings limited to the distal ileum. These include narrowing of the terminal ileum with discrete submucosal nodules measuring between 0.25 and 0.75 cm.

The colon may be variably involved. CT may reveal thickening of the wall of the distal ileum with associated colonic disease. Small-bowel obstruction may result from the transmural process.

Neoplasms

KS and NHL account for neoplastic complications in the small bowel of AIDS patients.

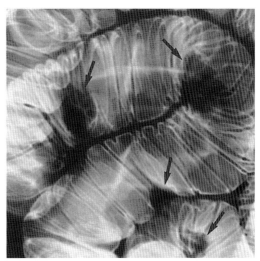

Fig. 13.**12** KS of the small bowel (enteroclysis). Multiple submucosal nodules (arrows) on normal intervening mucosa of the jejunum

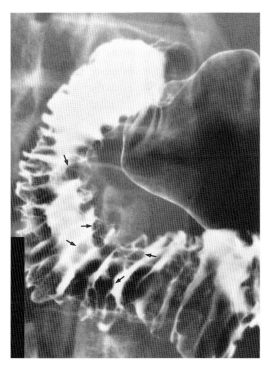

Fig. 13.**11** KS of the duodenum; thickening of mucosal folds with submucosal nodules scattered throughout the duodenum (arrows)

Kaposi's Sarcoma

KS lesions present as discrete submucosal nodules (48, 74). They generally vary in size from 1 to 2 cm (Fig. 13.11). Preservation of mucosal folds between the lesions distinguishes KS lesions from nodules of lymphoma which are associated with diffuse submucosal infiltration of the bowel wall (Fig. 13.**12**). When the caliber and fold pattern of the small bowel are distorted, one must consider such complications of KS as intramural hemorrhage or coexistent lymphoma in the differential diagnosis.

The small-bowel series is relatively insensitive to KS lesions. Careful fluoroscopy-guided spot filming using graded compression may be necessary to demonstrate the lesions that may be hidden between folds. Diffuse fold thickening can not be differentiated from lymphoma. Differentiation is possible with endoscopy that can depict su-

perficial incipient lesions represented by small macular mucosal discoloration (74, 75). KS rarely causes complications in the small bowel. Anecdotal cases of KS lesions leading to intussusceptions have been described. These lesions rarely bleed unless the patient is on an anticoagulant therapy or has a bleeding diathesis.

Non-Hodgkin's Lymphoma

Lymphoma may involve the small bowel, producing a variety of radiographic appearances. In our experience, focal lesions with discrete, penetrating ulcers or multiple nodules with associated bowel thickening are the most common radiographic appearances in AIDS-related lymphoma. As stated previously, unlike classic GI lymphoma, AIDS-related GI lymphoma is more commonly seen distal to the ligament of Treitz (Figs. 13.**13**, 13.**14**).

CT scanning has a high sensitivity in detection of GI lymphoma (76) and is the imaging modality of choice to exclude this diagnosis in AIDS patients (43, 62; Fig. 13.**15**). Findings include variably thickened small bowel loops with loss of mucosal

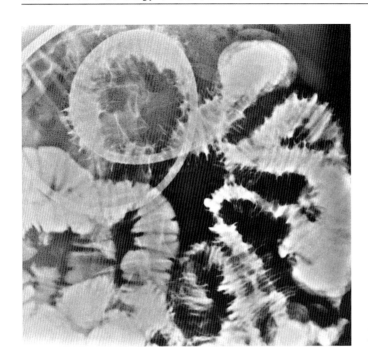

Fig. 13.**13** AIDS-related B-cell lymphoma of the proximal small bowel; thickening of folds, fixation, and mesenteric infiltration

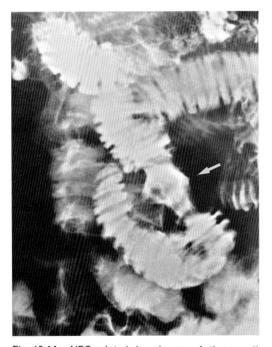

Fig. 13.**14** AIDS-related lymphoma of the small bowel

features resulting in blunted folds. As opposed to classic small-intestinal lymphoma, mesenteric adenopathy is infrequently visualized.

Colon

Nonneoplastic Lesions

Colitis

Colitis due to a variety of organisms is prevalent in the gay population. Many individuals harbor herpes, amebae, gonococci, shigellae, salmonellae, *Campylobacter*, *Candida*, and *Giardia*. The gay bowel syndrome has been described as being due to a variety of common pathogens (8, 33, 77; Fig. 13.**16**). These patients may also have a variety of anal infections. Nonspecific periproctitis may be visualized in CT scanning as a hazy increased density in the perianal fat (Table 13.**4**). Moon et al. (78) described perirectal abnormalities in 23 of 28 (82%) homosexual men with AIDS-related KS and lymphadenopathy syndrome. In 22 of 23, abnormalities were due to inflammatory disease rather than tumor. Albin et al. (79) reported rectal and perirectal abnormalities visualized by CT in 8 of 30 patients. In this series, 6 of 8 had inflammatory disease and 2 had tumor. The CT appearances were identical in both groups. Several colitides are unique in AIDS patients. Only CMV colitis produces radiographic findings that may be distinguishable from other infectious colitides (Table 13.5). Cryptosporidia and MAI infections have been documented in the colon of AIDS patients, but they do not produce characteristic X-ray findings. In Wall's series (11), 16 of 19 patients had an abnormal barium enema. All segments of the colon were equally involved.

In the series by Frager et al. (2), five patients demonstrated colonic disease, all due to CMV infection.

CMV Colitis

CMV colitis may be mild, or there may be fulminant disease leading to toxic megacolon, gangrenous necrosis of the bowel wall (30, 32, 70, 71, 80). Hemorrhagic colitis may be seen. The predilection of cecal involvement with multiple, deep linear ulcers as seen in renal transplant patients is also seen in the AIDS population (81).

The colon is the most frequent site of CMV-1B infection in AIDS patients. As compared with other immunosuppressed patients, those with AIDS have higher titers to CMV-1B and the colon is more frequently involved than the upper GI tract. CMV may be more easily cultured from the right colon than from the sigmoid colon (82).

Balthazar et al. (26) described the radiographic findings in 11 patients with CMV colitis. In 8 positive cases studied by barium enema, 3 showed diffuse mucosal granularity involving the entire colon. One patient

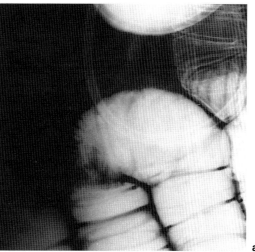

a

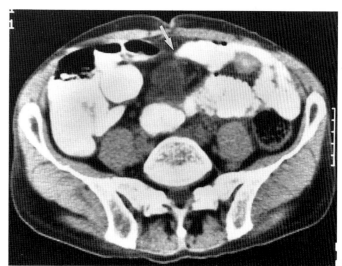

b

Fig. 13.**15** Enteroclysis (**a**): focal AIDS-related lymphoma in the proximal jejunum, better visualized on CT (**b**)

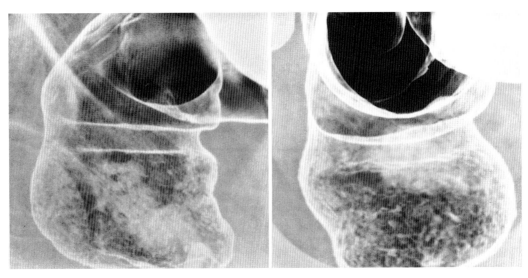

Fig. 13.**16**   Gonorrheal proctitis (gay bowel syndrome)

Table 13.**4**   Spectrum of radiologic features of the proctocolon in gay bowel syndrome

Organism/disease	Radiologic features	Extent of disease

Gay bowel syndrome
  N. gonorrhea
  Herpes simplex
  Chlamydia trachomatis
  (lymphogranuloma venereum)
  Entamoeba histolytica
  Salmonella
  Shigella
  Campylobacter
  Candida
  Giardia
	Edema with thumbprinting
	Diffuse (shallow) ulcerations
	  (collar buttons)
	Mucosal granularity
	Spasm, loss of distensibility
	Widening of presacral space
	Narrowing of the lumen
	CT Hazy increased density
	  in perianal fat
		Segmental or diffuse

showed involvement of the left colon. In 4 cases, cecal spasm with ulceration and terminal ileal fold effacement is present. Frager et al. (3) reported a spectrum of radiographic changes from a mild reticular, granular mucosal pattern with aphthous ulcers (Fig. 13.**17**) to multiple large discrete ulcers (Fig. 13.**18**) and submucosal hemorrhage in severe cases.

Barium enema is infrequently used to diagnose CMV colitis, ultrasound (Fig. 13.**19**) and endoscopy are utilized in symptomatic individuals (28). In those with unclear symptomatology, CT scanning is the primary imaging modality (19, 83). Findings include thickening of the colonic wall (Fig. 13.**20**) and a "target" pattern due to submucosal edema. Most cases show a pancolitis, but right-sided involvement is always present. Sometimes associated thickening of the wall of the distal ileum is noted. Contiguous involvement of the ileum and right colon, associated "target" pattern, and variable distal colitis may be considered virtually diagnostic of CMV colitis in an AIDS patient. In advanced stages, patients with CMV colitis may present with toxic dilatation of the colon often progressing to perforation. Plain films reveal a dilated colon with detectable nodularity along the wall. CT shows a thin-

Table 13.5 Spectrum of radiologic features in AIDS of the colon

Organism/disease	Radiologic features	Extent of disease
Nonneoplastic lesions		
CMV	*Mild*	Segmental or diffuse
	Diffuse mild or coarse mucosal granularity	Predilection for the right colon
	Cecal spasm	
	Irregular thickening of mucosal folds (edema)	
	Superficial or deep punctate or linear ulcerations	
	Aphtous ulcers	
	Fulminant	
	Large ulcers	
	Skip lesions	
	Areas of mass effect (granulation tissue/submucosal hemorrhage)	
	Nodular filling defects (pseudomembranes)	
	Toxic megacolon	
	Intramural gas dissection	
	Perforation	
	Late stage	
	Narrowing of the lumen	
	CT Thickening of colonic wall	
	"Target" pattern (submucosal edema)	
	Associated thickening of the distal ileum wall	
Neoplasms		
Kaposi's sarcoma	Localized clusters of undulating filling defects	Focal or diffuse
	Granular focal plaque-like lesions	
	Normal intervening mucosa	
	Narrowing of the lumen	
Non-Hodgkin's lymphoma	Polypoid lesions, simulating adenocarcinoma	Focal
	Bulky mass	Predilection for the rectum
	Lymphadenopathy: infrequent	
	CT Discrete to infiltrating perianal/perirectal mass	
	Infiltration of pelvic floor	
	Lymphadenopathy: infrequent	

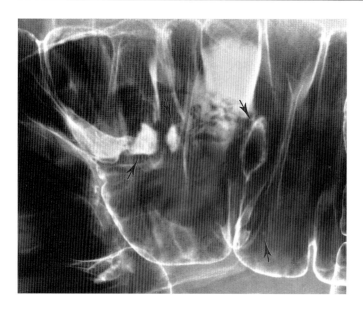

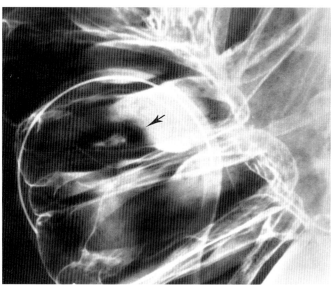

Fig. 13.**17**   CMV colitis; large aphthous ulcers with a halo (arrows) on normal mucosal background

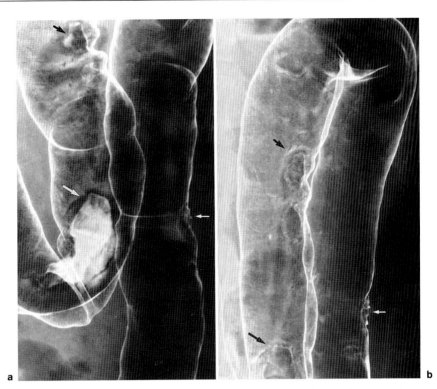

Fig. 13.**18** CMV colitis. Shallow, poorly defined oval and semilunar ulcers with a halo (arrows) on normal mucosal background; note the "diamond shaped" ulcer, 4 cm deep (small arrows), at the mid-part of the transverse colon (**a, b**)

walled colon and serosal enhancement. Intra-mural gas dissection may be visualized within the wall, indicative of vascular compromise. Peritoneal fluid is seen in association with the dilated colon and CMV organisms may be recovered from it. Occasionally patients may present with spontaneous pneumatosis coli. These findings result from the vasculitis induced by CMV inclusion bodies that may be found in the endothelial cells of the submucosal vessels and may lead to ischemic necrosis of the bowel wall.

Neoplasms

KS and lymphoma are the two major neoplasms found in the colon of AIDS patients.

Kaposi's Sarcoma

KS presents with either isolated submucosal plaques or focal areas of submucosal infiltration (Figs. 13.21, 13.22). This submucosal infiltration may be reflected as a localized cluster of undulating filling defects that narrows the colonic lumen, or as a granular focal plaque-like lesion along various segments of bowel.

Non-Hodgkin's Lymphoma

Colonic lymphoma is more common in the AIDS population than in non-AIDS patients with bowel lymphoma. Polypoid lesions simulating adenocarcinoma and bulky masses leading to intussusception have been seen (Figs. 13.23–26). There is a high pre-

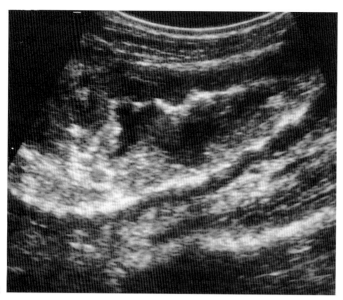

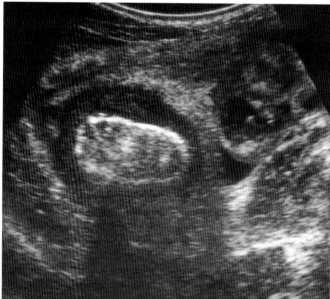

Fig. 13.**19** Sagittal (**a**) and transverse (**b**) scans on an HIV-positive patient with acute CMV typhlitis, histologically confirmed. Courtesy: S. R. Wilson, M.D., FRCP(C) The Toronto Hospital, Toronto, Canada

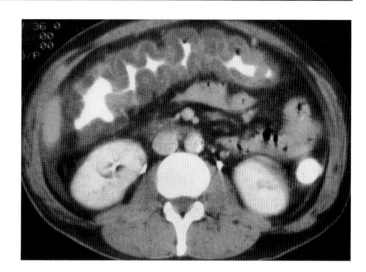

Fig. 13.**20** CMV colitis in AIDS; CT: thickening of the wall of the transverse colon

dilection for rectal involvement in AIDS-related lymphoma. Bulky infiltrating masses surrounding the rectum and infiltrating the pelvic floor and discrete perianal masses may be encountered. As in our cases of small-bowel lymphoma, there often is a striking lack of nodal disease in these patients.

Biliary Disease

Recent attention has been directed at involvement of the biliary tract in AIDS patients. Most reported cases described acalculous cholecystitis secondary to CMV or cryptosporidial infection (84, 85).

A recent report documented the radiographic findings in nine AIDS patients with right upper quadrant pain, jaundice, or abnormal liver function tests. Eight of the nine imaging studies disclosed intrahepatic or extrahepatic bile duct changes identical to those seen in sclerosing cholangitis. Isolated papillary stenosis in ductal dilatation was present in one patient. Eight patients had some stricturing of the distal common bile duct. Cholangitis caused by CMV or *Cryptosporidium* is the proposed pathogenic mechanism (29, 86).

In the series by Teixidor et al. (33), one patient was shown to have CMV infection of the biliary tree. The finding in this case was that of a stenosing papillitis. CMV and reovirus III have a tropism for bile duct epithelium in the neonate (85). Reflux of the organisms through the ampulla of Vater presumably when there is superinfection in the duodenum or small bowel may be responsible for this disorder.

In any AIDS patient with abnormal liver function tests, imaging generally will be performed to evaluate the presence of hepatomegaly or space-occupying lesions within the liver. Careful attention should be paid to the bile ducts. If segmental dilatation of any portion of the biliary tree is seen, direct cholangiography may be useful to document the presence of AIDS-related cholangitis. Ultrasonic visualization of gallbladder wall thickening, bile duct dilatation, and altered echogenicity in the periportal regions have been shown to be suggestive for AIDS-related cholangitis (87, 88).

Liver and Spleen

The reticuloendothelial elements in the liver and spleen may manifest radiographic abnormalities indicative of systemic infection. Recent reports of extrapulmonary PCP have described the presence of diffuse punctate calcifications as a manifestation of PCP granulomas in the organs (89, 90; Figs. 13.27, 13.28). Serial studies reveal that the lesion may initially appear as cysts which progressively and peripherally calcify. Calcification has been observed in the adrenals, kidneys (which demonstrate a peculiar cortical distribution), and peritoneal cavity. The almost simultaneous appearance of these patients in several centers which see a large number of AIDS patients suggests that this may be an epiphenomenon related either to a change in the PCP organism or perhaps an alteration of the host response to the organism induced by local control, specifically, with the increased availability of aerosolized pentamidine.

Lymphadenopathy

The presence of lymphadenopathy in AIDS patients may be secondary to a variety of causes. Most patients are referred to CT scanning because peripheral adenopathy is detected by physical examination. Persistent generalized lymphadenopathy is a component of AIDS-related complex. This benign reactive adenopathy is seen distributed within the retroperitoneum, the nodes being no greater than 1.5 cm in diameter (78, 91). When larger nodes are seen, or the nodes are within the small-bowel mesentery, other causes of adenopathy must be suspected.

Bulky adenopathy, mesenteric location, and occasional low-density areas within the nodes is characteristic of tuberculous adenitis. CT may be the first examination to suggest this diagnosis. This combination of findings was present in 82% of cases reported in one study (42). *Mycobacterium tuberculosis* or atypical forms such as MAI produce identical findings (Fig. 13.29).

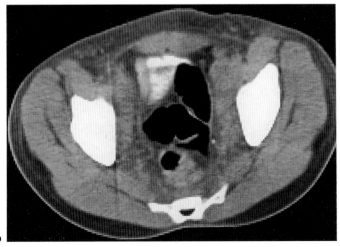

Fig. 13.21   KS of the rectum
a nodular filling defects in the proximal part of the rectum on DC study
b CT: contrast enhanced lesions on the dorsal/left side of the air-filled rectum

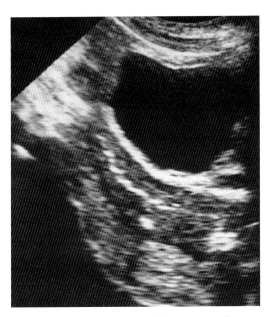

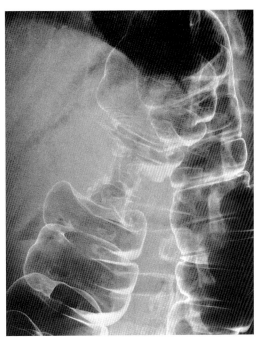

Fig. 13.**22** Ultrasonography of the rectum: disseminated Kaposi's sarcoma in the rectum in AIDS. Courtesy: S. R. Wilson, M.D., FRCP(C) The Toronto Hospital, Toronto, Canada

Fig. 13.**23** AIDS-related lymphoma; Circumscript stenotic lesion without shouldering at the distal transverse colon, simulating adenocarcinoma

Nodal disease secondary to KS may present as brightly enhancing nodes. On dynamic scans, these nodes may be as bright as the enhanced great vessels. In advanced cases, irregular margination reflects the predilection for soft-tissues infiltration.

AIDS-related lymphoma (ARL) tends to be extranodal. Gastrointestinal involvement is common, occurring in 22–33% of cases (62, 64, 92). The disease is seen more often distal to the ligament of Treitz as compared with "classic" bowel lymphoma. Nodal disease, when seen, is almost always pelvic in location and is usually of the Burkitt type. ARL is frequently present in solid organs presenting as focal masses within the liver (Fig. 13.**30**), spleen, and kidney. Peritoneal lymphomatosis has also been seen with increasing frequency in AIDS patients, although this complication is not exclusively seen in this group of patients (93).

Other neoplasms have also been reported in patients with AIDS: squamous cell carcinoma of the tongue, esophagus (54, 94), adenocarcinoma of the colon (Fig. 13.**31**), and cloacogenic carcinoma of the anus (80).

Pediatric AIDS

Pediatric AIDS accounts for 1.5% of the total cases of AIDS reported (95). Primarily two factors expose a child to the AIDS virus: maternal high risk situations (promiscuity, intravenous drug abuse) and blood transfusions.

The most common abdominal manifestations of pediatric AIDS is mesenteric and retroperitoneal lymphadenopathy (MAI) which may be the only imaging manifestation of AIDS, followed by hepatosplenomegaly as a nonspecific finding (96). NHL and KS,

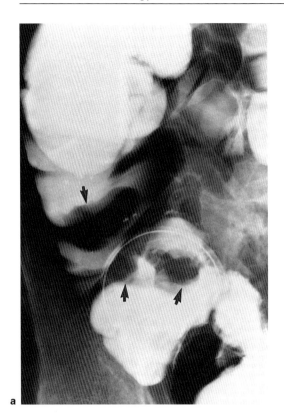

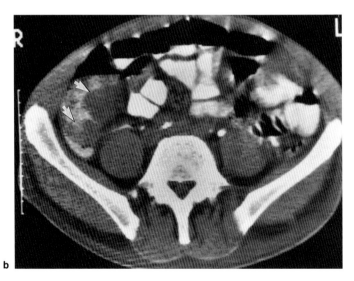

Fig. 13.**24** **a** Single-contrast barium enema. AIDS-related non-Hodgkin's lymphoma in the cecum at the level of Bauhin's valve. Nodular, sharply demarcated protrusions into the colonic lumen (arrows)
b CT: nodular protrusions into the bowel lumen (arrows)

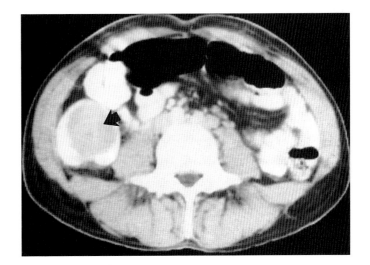

Fig. 13.**25** AIDS-related lymphoma. Large intraluminal soft tissue mass is seen in the ascending colon (arrow)

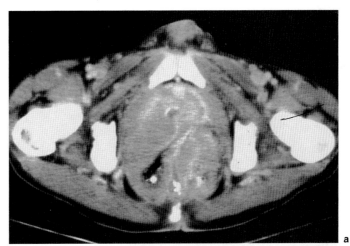

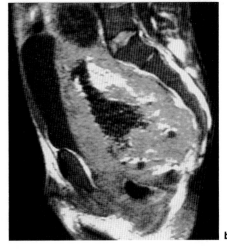

Fig. 13.**26** AIDS-related rectal lymphoma
a CT: circumferentially growing tumor mass which narrows the lumen
b MRI: T1 sagittal view

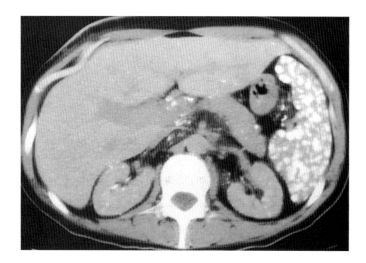

Fig. 13.**27**   Extrathoracic *Pneumocystis carinii* pneumonia. Discrete calcifications are seen in the spleen, liver, kidneys, and peripancreatic nodes

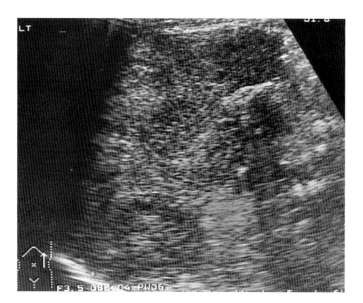

Fig. 13.**28**   Extrathoracic *Pneumocystis carinii* pneumonia. US: discrete calcifications are seen in the spleen (Courtesy N. J. Smits, M. D. Academic Medical Center, Amsterdam)

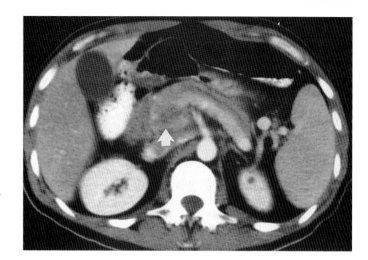

Fig. 13.**29** *M. tuberculosis.* Peripancreatic (hepatoduodenal
ligament) lymphadenopathy is
detected by CT in this patient
with fever of unknown origin

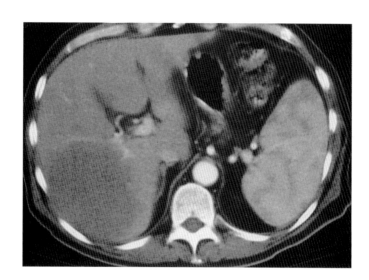

Fig. 13.**30**   AIDS-related lymphoma in the liver. Dynamic
CT scan reveals a homoge-
neously attenuating neoplasm
in the posterior right lobe

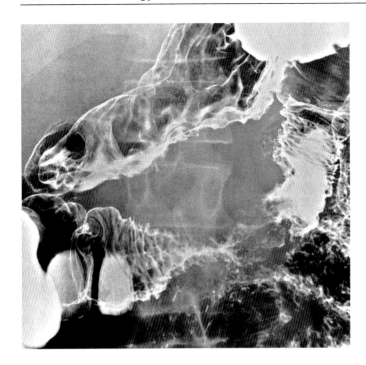

Fig. 13.**31** Simultaneous DC study of the stomach and colon: stenosis of the mid – colon transversum with serrations of the contour ("pleating sign"); irregular indentation of the large curvature of the stomach. Diagnosis: diffuse infiltrating adenocarcinoma of the colon in an AIDS patient

fairly common in adults with AIDS, are much less common in the pediatric AIDS group (95).

Children with KS do not have the skin and oral manifestations of the disease (97). The most common intrinsic gastrointestinal manifestations in pediatric AIDS is *Candida* esophagitis, with or without oral thrush. *Candida* esophagitis in a child who does not have a primary or secondary immunodeficiency is suggestive of AIDS (95). *Cryptosporidium*, HSV, and CMV infections may occur.

References

1. Centers for Disease Control. Revision of the CDC surveillance care definition for acquired immunodeficiency syndrome. MMWR 1987;62.
2. Frager DH, Frager JD, Brandt JL, et al. Gastrointestinal complications of AIDS: radiologic features. Radiology 1986;158:597–605.
3. Frager DH, Frager JD, Wolfe EL, et al. Cytomegalovirus colitis in acquired immune deficiency syndrome: radiologic spectrum. Gastrointest Radiol 1986;11:241–6.
4. Gottlieb MS, Groopman JE, Weinstein WM, Fahey JL, Detels R. The acquired immunodeficiency syndrome. Ann Intern Med 1983; 99: 208–20.
5. Jaffe HW, Bregman DJ, Selik RM. Acquired immune deficiency syndrome in the United States: the first one thousand cases. J Infect Dis 1983;148:339–45.
6. Landesman SH, Ginzburg HM, Weiss SH. Special report: the AIDS epidemic. N Engl J Med 1985;312:521–4.
7. Solinger AM, Hess EV. Acquired immune deficiency syndrome: an overview. Semin Roentgenol 1987;22:9–13.
8. Quin TC, Stamm WE, Goodell SE, et al. Polymicrobial origin of intestinal infections in homosexual men. N Engl J Med 1983;309:576–82.
9. Fauci AS. Acquired immune deficiency syndrome: an update. Ann Intern Med 1985; 102:800.
10. Federle MP. Radiologist looks at AIDS: imaging evaluation based on symptom complexes. Radiology 1988;196:553.
11. Wall SD, Ominsky S, Altman DF, et al. Multifocal abnormalities of the gastrointestinal tract in AIDS. AJR 1968;146:1–7.
12. Laufer I. Double contrast gastrointestinal radiology with endoscopic correlation. Philadelphia: WB Saunders, 1979.

13. Balthazar EJ, Megibow AJ, Hulnick DH, Cho C, Beranbaum ER. Cytomegalovirus esophagitis in AIDS: radiographic features in 16 patients. AJR 1987;149:919–25.

14. Farman J, Tavitian LE, Rosenthal GE, et al. Focal esophageal candidiasis in acquired immunodeficiency syndrome (AIDS). Gastrointest Radiol 1986;11:213–18.

15. Levine MS, lauder L, Kressel HY, Friedman H. Herpes esophagitis. AJR 1981;136:863–6.

16. Levine MS, Macones AJ Jr, Laufer I. *Candida* esophagitis: accuracy of radiographic diagnosis. Radiology 1985;154:581–7.

17. Levine MS, Woldenberg R, Herlinger H, Laufer I. Opportunistic esophagitis in AIDS: radiographic diagnosis. Radiology 1987;165:815–20.

18. Levine MS. Radiology of the esophagus. New York: WB Saunders, 1989.

19. Megibow AJ, Wall SD, Balthazar EJ. Rybak BJ. Gastrointestinal radiology in AIDS patients. In: Federle M, Megibow AJ, Naidich DP, eds. Radiology of AIDS. New York: Raven Press, 1988.

20. Alpern MB, Lawson TL, Foley WD, et al. Focal hepatic masses and fatty infiltration detected by enhanced dynamic CT. Radiology 1986;158:51.

21. Klein RS, Harris CA, Small CB. Oral candidiasis in high risk patients as initial manifestation of acquired immune deficiency syndrome. N Engl J Med 1984;311:354.

22. Roberts L, Gibbons G, et al. Adult esophageal candidiasis: a radiographic spectrum. Radiographics 1987;7:289.

23. Laufer I. Radiology of esophagus. Radiol Clin North Am 1982;20:687–99.

24. Goldberg H, Dodds WJ. Cobblestone esophagus due to monilial infection. AJR 1968;104:608.

25. Balthazar EJ, Megibow AJ, Hulnick DH. Cytomegalovirus esophagitis and gastritis in aquired immune deficiency syndrome. AJR 1985; 144:1201–4.

26. Balthazar EJ, Megibow AJ, Fazzini E, et al. Cytomegalovirus colitis: radiographic findings in 11 patients. Radiology 1985; 155:585–9.

27. Campbell DA, Piercey RA, Shnitka TK, Goldsand G, Devine RDO, Weinstein WM. Cytomegalovirus-accociated gastric ulcer. Gastroenterology 1977;72:533–5.

28. Cho S, Tisnado J, Liu C, Beachley MC, Shaw C, Kipreos BE, Schneider V. Bleeding cytomegalovirus ulcers of the colon: barium enema and angiography. AJR 1981;136:1213–15.

29. Galloway PG. Widespread cytomegalovirus infection involving the gastrointestinal tract, biliary tree and gallbladder in immuno-compromised patients. Gastroenterology 1984; 87:1407.

30. Knapp AB, Horst DA, Eliopoulos G, et al. Widespread cytomegalovirus gastroenterocolitis in a patient with acquired immune deficiency syndrome. Gastroenterology 1983;85:1399–1402.

31. Weinstein L, Edelstein SM, Madara JL, Falchuk KR, McManus BM, Trier JS. Intestinal cryptosporidiosis complicated by disseminated cytomegalovirus infection. Gastroenterology 1981;81:584–91.

32. Meiselman MS, Cello JP, Margareten W. Cytomegalovirus colitis in acquired immune deficiency syndrome. Gastroenterology 1985;88:171–5.

33. Teixidor HS, Honig CL, Norsoph E, Alberts S, Mouradian JA, Whalen JP. Cytomegalovirus infection of the alimentary canal: radiographic findings with pathologic correlation. Radiology 1987;163:317–25.

34. St Onge G, Bezahler GH. Giant esophageal ulcer associated with cytomegalovirus. Gastroenterology 1982; 83:127–30.

35. Agha FP, Horchang HL, Nostrant TT. Herpetic esophagitis: a diagnostic challenge in immunocompromised patients. Am J Gastroenterol 1986;81:246–53.

36. Shortsleeve MJ, Gauvin GP, Gardner RC, et al. Herpetic esophagitis. Radiology 1981;141:611–17.

37. Skucas J, Schrank WW, Meyers PC, et al. Herpes esophagitis: a case studied by air-contrast esophagography. AJR 1977;128:497–9.

38. Thoeni RF, Margulis AR. Gastrointestinal tuberculosis. Semin Roentgenol 1979;14:283–94.

39. Greene JR, Sidhu S, Lewin S, et al. *Mycobacterium avium–intracellulare*: a case of dissemination life-threatening infection in homosexual drug abusers. Am Intern Med 1982;97:539.

40. Goodman MD, Poster DD. Cytomegalovirus vasculitis with fatal colonic hemorrhage. Arch Pathol 1973;96:281–4.

41. Pitchenik AE, Cole C, Russell BW, Fischl MA, Spira TJ, Snider DE. Tuberculosis, atypical mycobacteriosis and the acquired immunodeficiency syndrome among Haitian and non-Haitian patients in South Florida. Ann Intern Med 1984;101:641–5.

42. Nyberg DA, Federle MP, Jeffrey RB, et al. Abdominal CT findings in disseminated *Mycobacterium avium–intracellulare*. AJR 1985;145:297–9.

43. Nyberg DA, Federle MP. AIDS-related Kaposi's sarcoma and lymphoma. Semin Roentgenol 1987; 22,I:54–65.

44. Goodman P, Pinero SS, Rance RM, Mansell DWA, Uribe-Botero G. Mycobacterial esophagitis in AIDS. Gastrointest Radiol 1989; 14:103–5.

45. Sohn CC, Schroff RW, Kliewer KE, Lebel DM, et al. Disseminated *Mycobacterium avium–intracellulare* infection in homosexual men with

acquired cell-mediated immunodeficiency: a histologic and pathologic study of two cases. Am J Clin Pathol 1983; 79:247.

46. Kaposi M. Idiopathisches multiples Pigmentsarkom der Haut. Arch Dermatol Syphilis 1872; 4:265–73.

47. Friedman-Kein AE, Laubenstein LJ, Rubinstein P, et al. Disseminated Kaposi's sarcoma in homosexual men. Ann Intern Med 1982; 96:693–700.

48. Hill CA, Harle TS, Mansell PWA. The procedure: Kaposi's sarcoma and infection associated with acquired immune deficiency syndrome, radiologic findings in 39 patients. Radiology 1983; 149:393–9.

49. Niedt GW, Schinella RA. Acquired immunodeficiency syndrome: clinicopathologic study of 56 autopsies. Arch Pathol Lab Med 1985; 109:727–34.

50. Longo DL. Kaposi's sarcoma and other neoplasms. Ann Intern Med 1984; 100:92–106.

51. Reed WB, Kamath HM, Weiss L. Kaposi's sarcoma with emphasis on the internal manifestations. Arch Dermatol 1974; 110:115–18.

52. Emery DC, Wall SD, Federle MP, Sooy CD. Pharyngeal Kaposi's sarcoma in patients with AIDS. AJR 1986; 147:919–22.

53. Lozada F, Silverman S, Conant M. New outbreak of oral tumors, malignancies, and infectious diseases strikes young homosexual. Can Dent Assoc J 1982; 10:30–42.

54. Lozada F, Silverman S, Migliorati CA, et al. Oral manifestations of tumor and opportunistic infections in the acquired immunodeficiency syndrome (AIDS): findings in 53 homosexual men with Kaposi's sarcoma. Oral Surg 1983; 56:491–4.

55. Ayulo M, Aisner SC, Margolis K, Moravex C. Cytomegalovirus-associated gastritis in a compromised host. JAMA 1980; 243:1364.

56. Dworkin B, Wormer GP, Rosenthal WS, et al. Gastrointestinal manifestations of acquired immune deficiency: a review of 22 cases. Am J Gastroenterol 1985; 80:774.

57. Brody JM, Miller DK, Zeman RK, et al. Gastric tuberculosis: a manifestation of AIDS. Radiology 1986; 159:347–8.

58. Federle MP, Nyberg DA, Hulnick DH, Jeffrey RB. Malignant neoplasms: Kaposi's sarcoma, lymphoma, and other diseases with similar radiologic features. In: Federle MP, Megibow A, Naidich DP, eds. Radiology of acquired immune deficiency syndrome. New York: Raven Press, 1988:107–29.

59. Cooper DA, Wodak A, Marriot DJ, et al. Cryptosporidiosis of the stomach and small intestine in patients in AIDS. Pathology 1984; 16:455–7.

60. Urba WS, Longo DL. Clinical spectrum of human retroviral induced diseases. Cancer Res 1985; 45:4637 s–43 s (suppl).

61. Ioachim FL, Cooper MC, Hellman GC. Lymphomas in men at high risk for acquired immunodeficiency syndrome (AIDS) Cancer 1985; 56: 2831–42.

62. Nyberg DA, Jeffrey RB, Federle MP, et al. AIDS-related lymphomas: evaluation by abdominal CT. Radiology 1986; 159:59–63.

63. Townsend RR, Laing FC, Jeffrey RB, Bottler K. Abdominal lymphoma in AIDS: evaluation with US. Radiology 1989; 171:719–24.

64. Ziegler JL, Beckstead JA, Volberding PA, et al. Non-Hodgkin's lymphoma in 90 homosexual men: relation to generalized lymphadenopathy. N Engl J Med 1984; 311:565–70.

65. Berg RN, Wall SD, McCardle GB, et al. Cryptosporidiosis of the stomach and small intestine in patients with acquired immune deficiency syndrome. AJR 1984; 143:549–54.

66. Gross TL, Wheat J, Bartlett M, O'Connor KW. AIDS and multisystem involvement with cryptosporidium. AMJ Gastroenterol 1986; 81:456–8.

67. Nime FA, Burek JD, Page D, et al. Acute enterocolitis in a human being infected with the protozoan Cryptosporidium. Gastroenterology 1987; 145:297–9.

68. Tzipori S, Smith M, Birch C, et al. Cryptosporidiosis in hospital patients with gastroenteritis. Am J Trop Med Hyg 1983; 32:9341–4.

69. Autran B, Gorin I, Leibowitch M. Acquired immune deficiency syndrome in a Haitian woman with cardic Kaposi's sarcoma and Whipple's disease. Lancet 1983; 1:767–8.

70. Frank D, Raicht RF. Intestinal perforation with CMV in patients with acquired immune deficiency syndrome. Am J Gastroenterol 1984; 79:201–5.

71. Gertler SC, Pressman J, Price P, et al. Gastrointestinal CMV infection in a patient with acquired immune deficiency syndrome. Gastroenterology 1983; 85:1399–402.

72. Roth R, Owen RL, Keven DF. Acquired immune deficiency syndrome with Mycobacterium avium–intracellulare lesions resembling those of Whipple's disease. N Engl J Med 1983; 309: 1324–35.

73. Vincent ME, Robbins AR. Mycobacterium avium–intracellulare complex enteritis: pseudo-Whipple's disease in acquired immune deficiency. AJR 1985; 144:921–2.

74. Rose HS, Balthazar EJ, Megibow AJ, et al. Alimentary tract involvement in Kaposi's sarcoma: radiographic and endoscopic findings in 25 homosexual men. AJR 1982; 139:661–6.

75. Weprin L, Zollinger R, Clausen KM, et al. Kaposi's sarcoma: endoscopic observations of gastric and colon involvement. J Clin Gastroenterol 1982; 4:357–360.

76. Megibow AJ, Balthazar EJ, Bosniak MA, Naidich DP. Computed tomography of gastrointestinal lymphoma. AMJ Roentgenol 1983; 141: 541–8.

77. Sider L, Mintzer RA, Mendelson EB. Radiologic findings of infection proctitis in gay men. AJR 1982;139:667–72.

78. Moon KL, Federle MP, Abrams DI, et al. Kaposi's sarcoma and lymphadenopathy syndrome: limitations of abdominal CT in acquired immunodeficiency syndrome. Radiology 1984; 150:479.

79. Albin J, Lewis E, Eftkhari F, Shirkhoda A. Computed tomography of rectal and perirectal disease in AIDS patients. Gastrointest Radiol 1987;12:67–71.

80. Cooper HS, Raffensperger EC, Jonas L. Cytomegalovirus inclusions in patients with ulcerative colitis and toxic dilatation requiring colonic resection. Gastroenterology 1977;72: 1253–6.

81. Foucar E, Mukai K, Foucan K, et al. Colon ulceration in lethal cytomegalovirus infection. Am J Clin Pathol 1981;76:788–801.

82. Hinnant K, Rotterdam HZ, Bell ET, Trapper ML. Cytomegalovirus infection of the alimentary tract: a clinicopathological correlation. Am J Gastroenterol 1986;81:944.

83. Megibow AJ. Gastrointestinal lymphoma: the role of CT in diagnosis and management. Semin Ultrasound CT MR 1986;7:43–57.

84. Kavin H, Jonas RB, Choudhury L, et al. Acalculous cholecystitis and cytomegalovirus infection in acquired immune deficiency syndrome. Ann Intern Med 1986;104:53–4.

85. Blumberg RS, Kelsey P, Perrone T, et al. Cytomegalovirus and cryptosporidia associated with acalculous cholecystitis. Ann J Med 1986;76:118–23.

86. Dolmatch BL, Laing FC, Federle MP, et al. AIDS-related cholangitis: radiographic findings in nine patients. Radiology 1987;163:313.

87. Romano AJ, van Sonnenberg E, Casola G, et al. Gallbladder and bile duct abnormalities in AIDS: sonographic findings in eight patients. AJR 1988;15:123.

88. Defalque D, Menu Y, Girard P, Couland J. Sonographic diagnosis of cholangitis in AIDS patients. Gastrointest Radiol 14:143.

89. Lubat E, Megibow AJ, Goldenberg A, Birnbaum BA, Balthazar EJ, Bosniak MA. Extrapulmonary *Pneumocystis carinii* infection in AIDS patients: CT findings. Radiology 1990;174:157–61.

90. Radin DR, Baker EL, Klatt EC, Balthazar EJ, Jeffrey RB, Megibow AJ, Ralls PW. Visceral and nodal calcifications in patients with AIDS-related *Pneumocystis carinii* infection. AJR 1990; 154: 27–31.

91. Jeffrey RB, Nyberg DA. Review: abdominal CT in AIDS: radiologic features. AJR 1986;146:7.

92. Abrams DI, Lewis BJ, Beckstead JH, et al. Persistent general lymphadenopathy in homosexual men: endpoint or prodrome. Ann Intern Med 1984;122:68.

93. Lynch MA, Cho KC, Jeffrey RB, et al. CT of peritoneal lymphomatosis. Am J Roentgenol 1988;151:715.

94. Frager DH, Wolfe EL, Competiello LS, Frager JD, Klein RS, Beneventano TC. Squamous cell carcinoma of the esophagus in patients with AIDS. Gastrointest Radiol 1988;13:358–60.

95. Amodio JB, Abramson S, Berdon WE, Levy J. Pediatric AIDS. Semin Roentgenol 1987; 22I: 66–76.

96. Abiri MM, Kirpekar M, Abiris S. The role of ultrasonography in the detection of extrapulmonary tuberculosis in patients with AIDS. J Ultrasound Med 1985;4:471–3.

97. Buck BE, Scott G, Dapena M, et al. Kaposi's sarcoma in 2 infants with AIDS. J Pediatr 1983; 103:911–13.

14 Nuclear Medicine Procedures in AIDS

E. A. van Royen

Introduction

The major advantage of nuclear medicine is its unique ability to detect functional and physiologic changes in disease that may procede the structural changes detectable by other imaging modalities. Nuclear medicine is an extremely versatile and flexible modality since an increasing number of radiolabeled chemical probes are being developed by modern chemical technology.

A disadvantage is the moderate quality of the images obtained, although the recent introduction of single photon emission computed tomography (SPECT) and new camera and computer developments are rapidly leading to an image much more appealing to the eye.

Infection by the human immunodeficiency virus is in theory an "ideal" disease to study with nuclear medicine techniques, because after the initial infection, there is a prolonged period with only subtle changes in immune function before the onset of macroscopic structural damage. During this period, patients in CDC classes I and II carry the virus asymptomatically, which may be identified by the presence of antibody. Serologic and immunologic study of peripheral blood samples can be used to monitor the progressive changes in immune functions at a high degree of reliability.

Up to now, little has been known of possible early, local changes in immune functions during this period. Ganz et al. (1) reported that, employing conventional technetium TC99m colloid spleen and liver scintigraphy early after infection, an increased spleen activity may be found. They attributed this phenomenon to an increased local phagocytosis, perhaps related to an activation of macrophages which has been suggested to occur before AIDS develops (2).

Future research may be directed into such local disarrangements employing labeled cells, monoclonal antibodies, or cellular products such as interferons or interleukins.

This review focuses on the value of nuclear medicine as a diagnostic method to detect infections, secondary malignancies, and neurologic disease in AIDS. Especially the role of gallium citrate Ga 67 scintigraphy in pulmonary disease and malignant lymphoma is stressed.

Gallium Citrate Ga 67

Gallium 67 was originally introduced as a bone-seeking radiopharmaceutical. Chemically it is a metal closely related to aluminium and iron, which is avidly bound by plasma transferrin after intravenous injection. The radionuclide ^{67}Ga has a half-life of 78 hours and disintegrates while emitting 3 gamma quanta of 93, 185, and 300 keV each. Although physically less ideal than ^{99m}Tc, it has relatively good properties for external imaging by gamma camera fitted with a medium energy collimator. A drawback is the limited possibility for SPECT imaging with ^{67}Ga.

Chemically the radionuclide is administered as citrate or chloride which is not critical for its target-seeking properties, since the gallium ion is bound to transferrin. The metalloprotein complex is retained in inflammatory tissue and many malignant tumours. The mechanism by which uptake and fixation of the tracer occur are not precisely understood. It usually takes 24 to 48 hours before images can be made.

The dose administered ranges from 40 to 400 MBq, depending on the aim of the study. For the demonstration of interstitial lung disease as in sarcoidosis, a low dose is sufficient, while for SPECT imaging of possible abdominal malignancies, higher doses are required.

Pneumocystis carinii pneumonia

PCP is the most common opportunistic infection in AIDS. It occurs as the initial manifestation in over 60% of the patients affected. The diagnosis depends on the demonstration of pneumocysts in ultrasonic nebulizer-induced sputum or more reliably by either bronchoalveolar lavage or transbronchial biopsy, or both. The sensitivity of the latter procedure is 90–95%, with a very high specificity.

Levenson et al. (3) described in the pre-AIDS era the abnormal accumulation of ^{67}Ga in the lungs of two patients infected with *P. carinii* after intensive chemotherapy for malignant lymphoma. The generalized pulmonary activity was markedly disproportionate to the clinical and radiologic findings and led to an earlier diagnosis by open lung biopsy.

Since then, numerous reports have been published on the high sensitivity and the lower specificity of ^{67}Ga scintigraphy to detect interstitial lung disease caused by *P. carinii* in AIDS patients (4–6). Also in this category of patients, PCP is characterized by a markedly increased, bilateral, diffuse uptake of the radionuclide in the lungs (Fig. 14.**1**). Normally little or no ^{67}Ga activity is measured in the lung area (Fig. 14.**2**). In our hospital, Reinders Folmer et al. (7) compared in a series of 11 patients the clinical findings, chest X-ray, CO transfer, and transbronchial biopsies or bronchoalveolar lavage with ^{67}Ga scintigraphy. They concluded that scintigraphy was a sensitive indicator of active disease, especially when the chest radiograph revealed no abnormality.

In a series of 34 patients, Barron et al. (6) reported an overall sensitivity of 94% and specificity of 74% of the scintigram to detect PCP as confirmed by transbronchial biopsy. The disease prevalence was about 50% in their group. If the chest X-ray was normal or equivocal, the sensitivity was 86% and the specificity 85%. Based on these data the

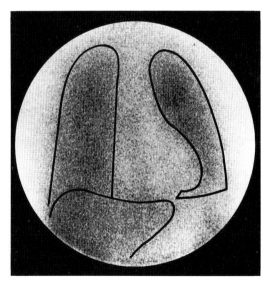

Fig. 14.**1** Markedly increased diffuse pulmonary uptake of ^{67}Ga in PCP infection in a 38-year-old man suffering from AIDS

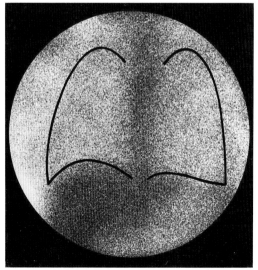

Fig. 14.**2** A normal ^{67}Ga scintigram of the thorax. There is little or no activity of the radionuclide found in the lung area. Notice the physiologic activity in liver and sternum

authors concluded that a negative scan is more reliable to exclude PCP than a positive scan to diagnose the disease.

The largest study conducted is by Kramer et al. (8). They evaluated 227 scans performed in a group of 180 HIV seropositive patients with a prevalence of PCP of 37% and compared the nuclear medicine results with those of chest X-ray and clinicopathologic diagnosis based on biopsy, culture, or response to specific therapy. The intensity of the ^{67}Ga uptake was graded on a scale of 0–4, grade 3 being an uptake intensity equal to and grade 4 greater than liver activity. Moreover, they characterized the uptake pattern as diffuse, focal extrapulmonary, focal intrapulmonary or ill-defined perihilar activity. In the case of a diffuse uptake, a distinction was made between homogeneous uptake and heterogeneous diffuse uptake.

They concluded that especially a heterogeneous intense uptake had an 87% positive predictive value for PCP. The positive predictive value of increased pulmonary activity for pathology of the lung was 93%, while a negative scan had a negative predictive value of 96%. If the intensity of lung uptake is less than liver uptake, the specificity falls to 50% due to other diffuse lung diseases, for example, CMV infection (see below).

Other Pulmonary Disorders

Increased pulmonary ^{67}Ga uptake is found in various other pathologic conditions frequently observed in AIDS. Cytomegalovirus (CMV) infection of the lung is characterized by a pattern of low-grade uptake with perihilar prominence (8; Fig. 14.3). Adrenal uptake due to CMV adrenalitis, which often comes along with CMV infection, may give a clue to this diagnosis on the ^{67}Ga scan (9). No larger series have been published on the sensitivity and specificity of this procedure.

Mycobacterium infection either by *M. tuberculosis* or *M. avium* accumulates ^{67}Ga avidly. Thadepalli et al. (10) described increased focal accumulation in lung and lymph nodes affected by active tuberculosis.

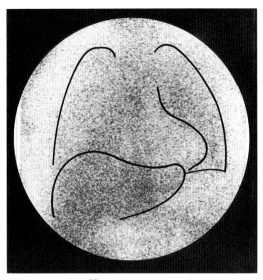

Fig. 14.3   Faint ^{67}Ga pulmonary activity in CMV infection in a 44-year-old AIDS patient

Following the publication of a case report of a diagnosis of disseminated *Mycobacterium* infection by ^{67}Ga in a patient suffering from AIDS (11), Kramer et al. (8) studied the efficacy in their large series. Nodal uptake suggested strongly *M. avium* or *tuberculosis*, especially if patchy lung activity is also found. Atypical mycobacterial infection presents more frequently with extra hilar nodes, while tuberculosis tends to be more commonly limited to hilar uptake (9). Malignant lymphoma and ARC lymphadenopathy (Fig. 14.4) with pure nodal activity have to be differentiated from *Mycobacterium* infection.

Figure 14.5 demonstrates the uptake of ^{67}Ga in tuberculosis.

Bacterial infections of the lung often show a pattern of localized lobar uptake of ^{67}Ga without nodal uptake. Lymphocytic interstitial pneumonitis (LIP) is a disorder of unknown etiology which is rare in adults with AIDS and relatively common in children. Zuckier et al. (12) described a 3-year-old child who demonstrated intense diffuse ^{67}Ga uptake due to LIP. Therefore, this condition can not be discerned from PCP based on the scintigraphic findings. A lower pulmonary uptake has been reported in adults with LIP (9), although supportive data are lacking.

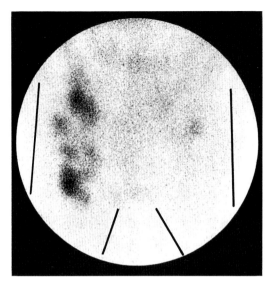

Fig. 14.**4** Gallium-67 uptake in ARC lymphadeno-pathy in the right inguinal area

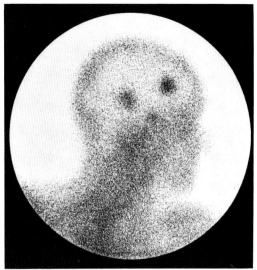

Fig. 14.**6** Gallium-67 uptake in malignant lym-phoma of the brain

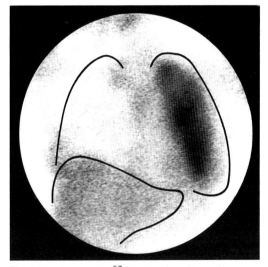

Fig. 14.**5** Intensive ^{67}Ga uptake in pulmonary tuberculosis of the left lung

Malignancies

Several reports confirm that Kaposi's sarcoma does not accumulate ^{67}Ga either in cutaneous (4), pulmonary (8), or mediastinal locations.

Thallium Tl 201 has been shown to accumulate in cutaneous, mucosal, and extra-cutaneous Kaposi lesions (13), like many other neoplastic lesions. Although it is a nonspecific uptake, in some conditions it may be of value to determine the extent of the disease. For the visualization of Kaposi's sarcoma, which are highly vascular tumors, ^{99m}Tc-labeled red blood cells have been suggested, but precise data are lacking.

Non-Hodgkin's lymphoma (NHL) has been recognized as an important sequela to AIDS. Apart from primary brain lymphoma (Fig. 14.**6**), high-grade NHL of B-cell origin is a frequent and serious manifestation of AIDS (14), generally with a poor prognosis. ^{67}Gallium scintigraphy, again, is an effective method of detecting site involvement in malignant lymphoma, especially if a higher dose (15) and SPECT (16) is applied. Especially during follow-up after therapy, ^{67}Ga scintigraphy is very useful and often superior to CT for detecting or excluding residual tumor or relapse.

Figure 14.**7** and Figure 14.**8** demonstrate the uptake of ^{67}Ga in 2 cases of AIDS-related malignant lymphoma.

Central Nervous System

Toxoplasma gondii is the most common cause of focal encephalitis in AIDS patients. Some

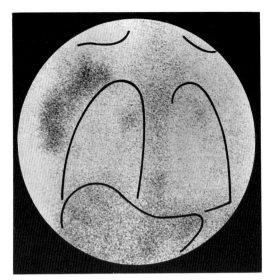

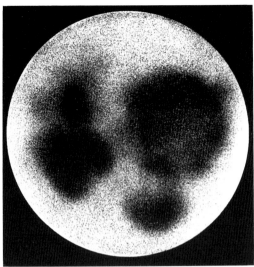

Fig. 14.**7** Gallium-67 accumulation in a case of AIDS-related malignant lymphoma located in the right axilla

Fig. 14.**8** Massive ^{67}Ga uptake in abdominal lesions of non-Hodgkin's lymphoma

role for indium In 111–labeled leukocyte scintigraphy in the diagnosis has been suggested (9), but little supportive data are available. Also in cryptococcal meningitis or CMV encephalitis the role of nuclear medicine procedures is limited.

A large percentage of patients may develop dementia due to the invasion of the brain tissue by the virus. It has been stated that nearly two-thirds of patients will eventually develop moderate to severe dementia (17). The brain tissue itself is, apart from the immunologic system, target to the retrovirus, which causes structural damage to the white matter and the deep gray nuclei, particularly the basal ganglia (18).

Characteristic alterations in regional cerebral glucose metabolism has been reported by Rottenberg et al. (19) employing positron emission tomography (PET) and fluorine F 18–labeled deoxyglucose. In early AIDS-related dementia, hypermetabolism in thalamus and basal ganglia occurred while later on, hypometabolism of cortical and subcortical gray matter dominated. The abnormalities of glucose metabolism have been shown to be reversible after azidothymidine (AZT) therapy (20).

Employing SPECT and a dopamine D_2-receptor ligand (iodine I 123–labeled IBZM), we were not able to find in a small series of AIDS patients any abnormality in D_2-receptor activity of the basal ganglia.

Regional cerebral blood flow (rCBF) in AIDS dementia has also been studied by SPECT. Patchy focal abnormalities were found (21) which differed from the bilateral temporo-occipital hypoperfusion in dementia of the Alzheimer type (22).

If structural brain damage is present, which will often be the case in these patients, for example, by toxoplasmosis or CMV, the rCBF images will be subject to nonspecific changes in affected areas, which is a drawback to a successful use of rCBF SPECT in this category of patients. No data on specificity and sensitivity in larger series are available.

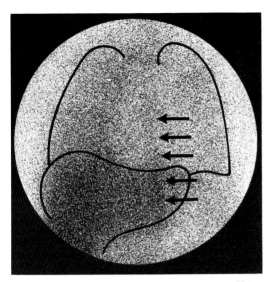

Fig. 14.**9** Increased pulmonary interstitial ^{67}Ga uptake due to PCP infection and increased midline activity over the esophageal area due to *Candida* esophagitis in a 30-year-old AIDS patient

Miscellaneous

Candida esophagitis may show up in the ^{67}Ga thoracic image as shown in Fig. 14.**9**, while CMV esophagitis does not.

Bone scintigraphy and ^{67}Ga scintigraphy are successful nuclear medicine procedures to demonstrate septic arthritis and osteomyelitis, which often occur with AIDS, days before radiographic abnormalities are found. AIDS-related myositis, a syndrome characterized by tenderness and weakness of the involved muscle groups, may be visualized on a ^{99m}Tc bone scintigraphy by extraosseous deposition of the diphosphonate in the affected muscles (23).

References

1. Ganz WI, Heiba A, Ganz SS, et al. Use of liver spleen scintigraphy to detect immune status and Kaposi's sarcoma in AIDS patients. Radiology 1987; 165:(P)97.
2. Fuchs D, Hausen A, Hengster P, et al. In vivo activation of CD4$^+$ cells in AIDS. Science 1987;235:356.
3. Levenson SM, Warren RD, Richman SD, et al. Abnormal pulmonary gallium accumulation in *P. carinii* pneumonia. Radiology 1976;119: 395–8.
4. Woolfenden JM, Carrasquillo JA, Larson SM, et al. Acquired immunodeficiency syndrome: Ga-67 imaging. Radiology 1987;162:383–7.
5. Bitran J, Bekerman C, Weinstein R, et al. Patterns of gallium-67 scintigraphy in patients with acquired immunodeficiency syndrome and the AIDS-related complex. J Nucl Med 1987; 28:1103–6.
6. Barron TF, Birnbaum NS, Shane LB, et al. Pneumocystis carinii pneumonia studied by gallium-67 scanning. Radiology 1985;154:791–3.
7. Reinders Folmer SCC, Danner SA, Bakker AJ, et al. Gallium-67 lung scintigraphy in patients with acquired immune deficiency syndrome (AIDS). Eur J Respir Dis 1986;68:313–18.
8. Kramer EL, Sanger JH, Garay SM, et al. Diagnostic implications of Ga-67 chest scan patterns in human immunodeficiency virus-seropositive patients. Radiology 1989;170:671–6.
9. Ganz WI, Serafini AN. The diagnostic role of nuclear medicine in the acquired immunodeficiency syndrome. J Nucl Med 1989;30:1935–45.
10. Thadepalli H, Rambhata K, Mishkin FS, et al. Correlation of microbiologic findings and ^{67}Gallium scans in patients with pulmonary infections. Chest 1977;72:442–8.
11. Malhotra C, Erickson AD, Feinsilver SH, et al. GA-67 studies in a patient with acquired immunodeficiency syndrome and disseminated mycobacterial infection. Clin Nucl Med 1985; 10:96–8.
12. Zuckier LS, Ongseng F, Goldfarb CR. Lymphocytic interstitial pneumonitis: a cause of pulmonary Gallium-67 uptake in a child with acquired immunodeficiency syndrome. J Nucl Med 1988;29:707–11.
13. Lee VW, Rosen MP, Baum A, et al. AIDS-related Kaposi's sarcoma: findings on Thallium-201 scintigraphy. Am J Radiol 1988; 151:1233–5.
14. Ziegler JL, Beckstead JA, Volberding PA, et al. Non-Hodgkin lymphoma in 90 homosexual men. New Engl J Med 1984;311:565–70.
15. Anderson KC, Leonard RCF, Canellos GP, et al. High-dose gallium imaging in lymphoma. Amer J Med 1983;75:327–31.
16. Tumeh SS, Rosenthal DS, Kaplan WD, et al. Lymphoma: evaluation with Ga-67 SPECT. Radiology 1987;164:111–14.
17. Navia BA, Jordan BD, Price RW. The AIDS dementia complex: I. clinical features. Ann Neurol 1986;19:517–24.
18. Navia BA, Cho ES, Petito CK, et al. The AIDS dementia complex: II. neuropathology. Ann Neurol 1986;19:525–35.

19. Rottenberg DA, Moeller JR, Strother SC, et al. The metabolic pathology of the AIDS dementia complex. Ann Neurol 1987;22:700–6.
20. Brunetti A, Berg G, DiChiro G, et al. Reversal of brain metabolic abnormalities following treatment of AIDS dementia complex with 3'-azido-2',3'-dideoxythymidine (AZT, Zidovudine): a PET-FDG study. J Nucl Med 1989;30:581–90.
21. Pohl P, Vogl G, Fill H, et al. Single photon emission computed tomography in AIDS dementia complex. J Nucl Med 1988;29:1382–6.
22. Weinstein HC, Hijdra A, van Royen EA, et al. Determination of cerebral blood flow by SPECT: a valuable tool in the investigation of dementia? Clin Neurol Neurosurg 1989;91:13–19.
23. Scott JA, Palmer EL, Fischman AJ. HIV-associated myositis detected radionuclide bone scanning. J Nucl Med 1989;30:556–8.

Index